Workbook for

Pilbeam's Mechanical Ventilation:

Physiological and Clinical Applications

Sixth Edition

Workbook for

Pilbeam's Mechanical Ventilation:

Physiological and Clinical Applications

Sixth Edition

Sandra T. Hinski

James M. Cairo

ELSEVIER

ELSEVIER

3251 Riverport Lane
Maryland Heights, MO 63043

WORKBOOK FOR PILBEAM'S MECHANICAL VENTILATION: ISBN: 9780323320986
PHYSIOLOGICAL AND CLINICAL APPLICATIONS

Content Strategist: Sonya Seigafuse
Content Development Manager: Billie Sharp
Content Development Specialist: Charlene Ketchum
Publishing Services Manager: Hemamalini Rajendrababu
Project Manager: Sukanthi Sukumar
Cover Designer: Gopalakrishnan Venkataraman

Working together
to grow libraries in
developing countries

www.elsevier.com • www.bookaid.org

Printed in the United States of America

Last digit is the print number: 9   8   7   6   5   4

To my husband Bill and my children Charlie and Stella, for their tolerance of the long days and nights I spent in my office writing. I love you and thank you. And to all my students for unknowingly pushing me to never stop learning.

Sandra T. Hinski

Preface

The goal of this workbook is to assist the respiratory care student in the mastery of the information presented in *Pilbeam's Mechanical Ventilation: Physiological and Clinical Applications,* Sixth Edition, by James M. Cairo.

Reading any medical textbook requires active participation, which is very different from the passive reading we do for pleasure. The reader should expect to read the material slowly and carefully to aid in the comprehension of the material. You should focus your attention on the information being presented. Reading with a purpose increases concentration, comprehension, retention, and interest in the subject matter.

I recommend that the student use the text and workbook in the following manner:

First, preview or scan through the text by reading the title, outline, objectives, and key terms. Remember: the learning objectives indicate what the author intends for the reader to know after finishing with the chapter. Skim the headings and subheadings. Read the Chapter summary. This highlights the structure of the chapter and emphasizes important concepts.

Next, turn the title into a question. The idea here is that asking a question focuses your reading on finding information that will help you answer the question. It makes reading a more active search for meaning. Use the review questions in the workbook to help you focus on important points in the chapter. Read carefully (in manageable chunks) to answer these questions. Note important details and relationships of ideas. The review questions in this workbook are based on the author's learning objectives for each chapter. Pay particular attention to the figures, boxes, tables, key points, case studies, and clinical scenarios because they are included to help learn the material.

Then review the textbook's Chapter Review Questions. Be able to answer all of the questions. This will ensure that highlighting or annotating the textbook is being done efficiently.

After this, answer the Critical Thinking Questions and the Case Study Questions in the Workbook. This will help with analysis and application-type questions seen on the board exams. Re-read any topic you are struggling with to ensure your understanding of the concept. The next step is to attempt the NBRC-type questions. Once you have read a chapter or topic, try reading peer-reviewed literature on the subject that includes experiments and case studies. This will help you apply your reading into the real world of respiratory care. And never forget to ask for help sooner rather than later if a topic is just not sinking in. ***All Answers for the Workbook are available through your Instructor via the Evolve website.***

Sandra T. Hinski, M.S., RRT-NPS

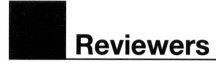

Reviewers

Allen Barbaro, MS, RRT
Department Chairman, Respiratory Care Education
St. Lukes College
Sioux City, Iowa

Richard Wettstein, MEd
Director of Clinical Education
University of Texas Health Science Center at San Antonio
San Antonio, Texas

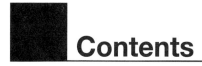

Contents

Basic Terms and Concepts of Mechanical Ventilation

LEARNING OBJECTIVES

On completion of this chapter the reader will be able to do the following:

1. Define *ventilation, external respiration,* and *internal respiration.*
2. Draw a graph showing how intrapleural and alveolar (intrapulmonary) pressures change during spontaneous ventilation and during a positive pressure breath.
3. Define the terms *transpulmonary pressure, transrespiratory pressure, transairway pressure, transthoracic pressure, elastance, compliance,* and *resistance.*
4. Provide the value for intra-alveolar (P_{alv}) pressure throughout inspiration and expiration during normal, quiet breathing.
5. Write the formulas for calculating compliance and resistance.
6. Explain how changes in lung compliance affect the peak pressure measured during inspiration with a mechanical ventilator.
7. Describe how changes in airway conditions can lead to increased resistance.
8. Calculate the airway resistance (R_{aw}) given the peak inspiratory pressure (PIP), a plateau pressure ($P_{plateau}$), and the flow rate.
9. From a figure showing abnormal compliance or airway resistance, be able to determine which lung unit will fill more quickly or with a greater volume.
10. Compare several time constants and explain how different time constants will affect volume distribution during inspiration.
11. Give the percentage of passive filling (or emptying) for one, two, three, and five time constants.
12. Briefly discuss the principle of operation of negative pressure, positive pressure, and high-frequency mechanical ventilators.
13. Define *peak inspiratory pressure, baseline pressure, positive end-expiratory pressure* (PEEP), and *plateau pressure.*
14. Describe the measurement of plateau pressure.

1

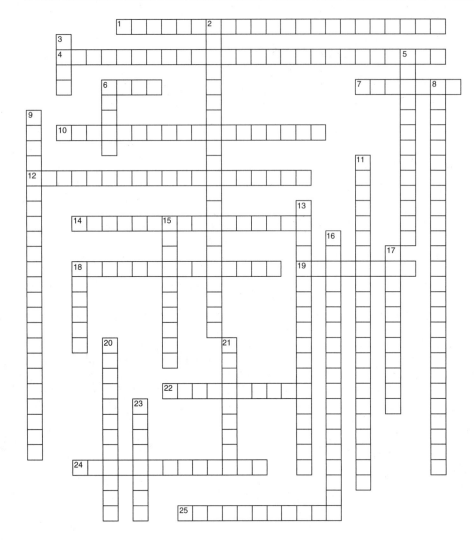

Across

1 Alternate term for pressure in the airways of the lungs (three words)
4 Total amount of gas remaining in the lungs after a resting expiration (three words)
6 Abbreviation for a form of ventilatory support characterized by rates up to 4000 breaths/min
7 Pressure measurement when there is no gas flow
10 Pressure measured in the esophagus that is used to represent intrapleural pressure (two words)
12 Movement of oxygen into cells and of carbon dioxide out of cells (two words)
14 Measurement of elastic forces that oppose lung inflation (two words)
18 Pressure in the airways of the lungs (two words)
19 Another term for intrinsic PEEP (hyphenated word)
22 Impedance of gas flow through the conductive airways
24 Deliberate increase in the ventilator's baseline pressure (two words)
25 Movement of gas molecules across a membrane

Down

2 Pressure measured at the mouth (three words)
3 Abbreviation for ventilation using small pulses of pressurized gas at rates between 100 and 400 breaths/min
5 Complication of positive pressure ventilation that causes an inadvertent buildup of positive pressure in the alveoli (two words)
6 Abbreviation for ventilation using lower than normal tidal volumes and respiratory rates between 60 and 100 breaths/min
8 Pressure between the alveolus and the pleural space responsible for maintaining alveolar inflation (three words)
9 Another term for the highest pressure recorded at the end of inspiration (three words)
11 Airway communications between the lung and pleural space (two words)
13 Highest pressure recorded at the end of inspiration (three words)
15 The ease with which the lungs distend
16 Movement of oxygen into the bloodstream and carbon dioxide out of the bloodstream (two words)
17 Movement of air into the lungs for gas exchange and out of the lungs for carbon dioxide removal
18 Functional unit of the lung
20 Mathematical expression used to describe the filling and emptying of lung units (two words)
21 Tendency of the lungs to return to their original form after being stretched
23 Difference between an area of high pressure and low pressure

CHAPTER REVIEW QUESTIONS

1. Describe the difference between ventilation and respiration.

   _____

   _____

   _____

   _____

2. The movement of oxygen and carbon dioxide in and out of the alveolar capillaries is known as _____, whereas the movement of oxygen and carbon dioxide in and out of body tissues is called _____

3. Describe the conditions necessary for air to flow from Point A to Point B in Figure 1-1.

   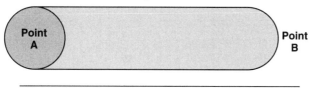

   _____

   _____

4. The pressure in the potential space between the parietal and visceral pleura is known as _____. At the end of exhalation during spontaneous breathing this pressure is approximately _____ and at the end of inspiration is about _____.

   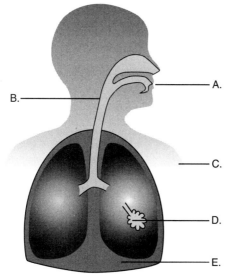

5. Use Figure 1-2 for this question.

   a. Identify the pressures labeled *A* through *E*.

   _____

b. Name at least three additional terms for pressure *A*.

   1. _____

   2. _____

   3. _____

6. How is intrapleural pressure (P_{pl}) estimated?

   _____

   _____

7. The pressure gradient between airway pressure and alveolar pressure is known as _____. This pressure is responsible for the movement of air in the _____. This gradient is calculated by the formula _____

8. The pressure needed to expand or contract both the lungs and the chest wall at the same time is _____. This pressure gradient is calculated by the formula _____

9. The pressure that is responsible for maintaining alveolar inflation is known as _____ and is calculated by the formula _____

10. The pressure that is required for inflation of the lungs and airways during positive pressure ventilation is called _____ and is calculated by the formula _____

11. Use Figure 1-2 to answer questions a through d.

    a. What pressure gradient is represented by Point A to Point C? What is its function during breathing?

    _____

    _____

    b. What pressure gradient is represented by Point C to Point D? What is its function during breathing?

    _____

    _____

    c. What pressure gradient is represented by Point D to Point E? What is its function during breathing?

    _____

    _____

d. What pressure gradient is represented by Point B to Point D? What is its function during breathing?

_____

_____

12. On the graph in Figure 1-3, label the *x*- and *y*- axes, draw the changes in P_alv during a spontaneous breath, and label inspiration and expiration.

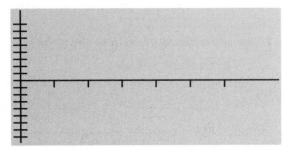

13. Describe how a negative pressure ventilator causes air to move into an individual's lungs.

_____

_____

_____

_____

14. List three advantages of using negative pressure ventilators.

   1. _____

   2. _____

   3. _____

15. Calculate the transairway pressure (P_{TA}) when the mouth pressure (P_M) is +25 cm H_2O and the P_{alv} is +5 cm H_2O.

_____

16. Draw and label, on the graph in Figure 1-4, the changes in intrapulmonary pressure that occur during a positive pressure breath with a PIP of 30 cm H_2O, a $P_{plateau}$ of 20 cm H_2O, PEEP of 5 cm H_2O, inspiratory time of 2 seconds, and expiratory time of 4 seconds.

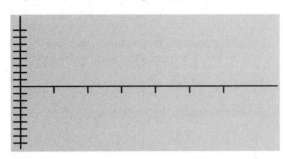

17. Draw and label, on the graph in Figure 1-5, the changes in intrapulmonary pressure that occur during a positive pressure breath with a PIP of 45 cm H_2O, a $P_{plateau}$ of 25 cm H_2O, PEEP of 10 cm H_2O, inspiratory time of 1 second, and expiratory time of 2 seconds, followed by a spontaneous breath with the same baseline.

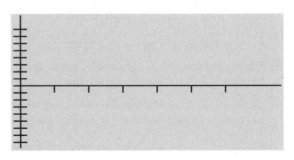

18. The highest pressure recorded at the end of inspiration is called _____ or

_____.

19. The pressure at which expiration ends is called

_____.

20. When end expiratory pressure is above atmospheric pressure, this is called _____.

21. The pressure required to overcome the elastic recoil of the lungs is known as _____ and is measured on a mechanically ventilated person by _____.

22. What are the two types of forces that oppose inflation of the lungs? _____ and _____

23. The relative ease with which a structure distends is known as _____, and the tendency of a structure to return to its original form after being stretched is known as _____.

24. Pulmonary compliance is defined as _____, and the formula is written as _____

25. Normally, total compliance of the lungs and thorax is about _____, but it can range from _____ to _____.

26. While mechanically ventilated, the compliance value for a male with normal lungs is _____ and for a female with normal lungs is _____.

27. What is the formula used to calculate static compliance?

_____

28. When more pressure is required to deliver a set tidal volume (V_T), what is likely happening to compliance?

_____

29. Calculate the static compliance when $P_{plateau}$ is 27 cm H_2O, baseline pressure is 10 cm H_2O, and V_T is 750 mL.

_____

30. Calculate the static compliance when $P_{plateau}$ is 35 cm H_2O, baseline pressure is 5 cm H_2O, and V_T is 575 mL.

_____

31. Calculate the static compliance when $P_{plateau}$ is 18 cm H_2O, baseline pressure is 0 H_2O, and V_T is 650 mL.

_____

32. What happens to PIP as the lungs become more difficult to ventilate? What happens to lung compliance?

_____

33. Define *resistance*.

_____

34. What is the formula for airway resistance (R_{aw})?

_____

35. What is the normal resistance range for flow rates of 0.5 L/s?

_____

36. What lung disease causes both airway resistance and static compliance to increase?

_____

37. Calculate the P_{TA} when PIP is 27 cm H_2O and $P_{plateau}$ is 20 cm H_2O.

_____

38. How much pressure is needed to overcome airway resistance when PIP is 30 cm H_2O and $P_{plateau}$ is 20 cm H_2O?

_____

39. What is the normal amount of pressure lost to airway resistance when a patient has a properly sized endotracheal tube?

_____

40. Calculate R_{aw} for a ventilated patient with the following: PIP 48 cm H_2O, $P_{plateau}$ 30 cm H_2O, and a set flow rate of 40 L/min.

_____

_____

41. Calculate airway resistance for a ventilated patient with the following: PIP 25 cm H_2O, $P_{plateau}$ 15 cm H_2O, and a set flow rate of 60 L/min.

_____

42. Why are the characteristics of the lung not homogenous?

_____

_____

43. Compare the filling time and volume for a normal lung unit, a low compliance unit, and a unit with high airway resistance using the same driving pressure.

_____

_____

_____

_____

44. What factors contribute to resistance when breathing?

_____

_____

45. What clinical factors can increase airway resistance by decreasing the radius of the airways?

_____

_____

46. How many seconds will it take to allow 86% of the V_T to be exhaled when compliance is 25 mL/cm H_2O and resistance is 30 cm H_2O/L/s?

_____

_____

47. Calculate the time constant for a mechanically ventilated patient when the V_T is 600 mL, PIP is 30 cm H_2O, $P_{plateau}$ is 24 cm H_2O, and flow rate is 60 L/min, with no PEEP.

_____

_____

_____

_____

48. What percentage of passive filling occurs for 1, 2, 3, 4, and 5 time constants?

_____

_____

49. The time constant for patient #1 is 0.05 second; patient #2 is 3 seconds; and 0.5 second for patient #3. If the same filling pressure is used for each, which patient will receive the most volume during inspiration and why?

_____

_____

_____

50. Calculate the time constant for a compliance of 55 mL/cm H_2O and resistance of 6 cm H_2O/L/s.

_____

_____

51. What is the inspiratory time setting to allow 95% volume emptying for a patient with the time constant calculated in Question 50?

_____

52. Why do patients with increased airway resistance develop air trapping when ventilator rates are set too high?

_____

_____

53. Calculate the time constant for a mechanically ventilated patient when the V_T is 700 mL, PIP is 45 cm H_2O, $P_{plateau}$ is 18 cm H_2O, flow rate is 60 L/min, and PEEP is 5 cm H_2O.

_____

_____

_____

_____

54. Which of the two lung units represented in Figure 1-6 will receive more volume given the same amount of time for inspiration? Explain your answer.

_____

_____

_____

_____

_____

55. Which of the two lung units represented in Figure 1-7 will fill more quickly? Explain your answer.

_____

_____

_____

_____

CRITICAL THINKING QUESTIONS

1. When the PIP is 43 cm H_2O and the $P_{plateau}$ is 18 cm H_2O, how much pressure is required to overcome the resistance of the airways?

   _____

   _____

2. What time constants would you expect for a patient with Adult Respiratory Distress Syndrome?

   _____

   _____

3. Describe how emphysema causes lung units to have long time constants.

   _____

   _____

   _____

4. What time constants would you expect for a 30-week (gestational age) premature infant?

   _____

5. When measuring the $P_{plateau}$ on a patient receiving mechanical ventilation you observe a $P_{plateau}$ that is higher than the PIP. What is one explanation for this?

   _____

   _____

   _____

CASE STUDIES

Case Study 1

A respiratory therapist reviews the following information concerning an intubated patient being mechanically ventilated.

Time	PIP	$P_{plateau}$	V_T	Set Flow Rate	PEEP
0800	18 cm H_2O	10 cm H_2O	600 mL	45 L/min	5 cm H_2O
1000	24 cm H_2O	12 cm H_2O	600 mL	45 L/min	5 cm H_2O
1200	35 cm H_2O	11 cm H_2O	600 mL	45 L/min	5 cm H_2O

1. What is the P_{TA} at 0800, 1000, and 1200?

   _____

   _____

2. Calculate the R_{aw} at 0800, 1200, and 1200.

   _____

   _____

   _____

   _____

Chapter **1** **Basic Terms and Concepts of Mechanical Ventilation**

3. Calculate the static compliance at 0800, 1000, and 1200.

_____

_____

_____

_____

4. Calculate one time constant at 0800, 1000, and 1200.

_____

_____

_____

5. a. What caused the PIP to rise between 0800 and 1200?
   b. What problems will this cause when ventilating the patient?

_____

_____

_____

_____

Case Study 2

The following information is obtained from the flow sheet of an intubated patient being mechanically ventilated.

Time	PIP	$P_{plateau}$	V_T	Set Flow Rate	PEEP
1000	40 cm H_2O	28 cm H_2O	550 mL	40 L/min	0 cm H_2O
1200	47 cm H_2O	37 cm H_2O	550 mL	40 L/min	5 cm H_2O
1400	54 cm H_2O	43 cm H_2O	550 mL	40 L/min	7 cm H_2O
1600	45 cm H_2O	33 cm H_2O	450 mL	60 L/min	12 cm H_2O

1. Complete the table below.

Time	P_{TA}	R_{aw}	C_{STAT}	Time Constant
1000				
1200				
1400				
1600				

2. What is the source of the rising PIP between 1000 and 1400?

_____

_____

_____

3. What would be the minimum inspiratory time for this patient at 1600 hours?

_____

1. Calculate the static effective compliance during the delivery of a ventilator breath with 650 mL with a $P_{plateau}$ of 28 cm H_2O and a PEEP of 0.
   a. 0.04 cm H_2O/L
   b. 0.23 L/cm H_2O
   c. 23 mL/cm H_2O
   d. Not enough information is given

2. Calculate the R_{aw} for a patient receiving mechanical ventilation with a set V_T of 825 mL and a peak flow setting of 50 L/min when the PIP is 46 cm H_2O and the $P_{plateau}$ is 22 cm H_2O.
   a. 13.7 cm H_2O/L/s
   b. 26.5 cm H_2O/L/s
   c. 28.9 cm H_2O/L/s
   d. 38.2 cm H_2O/L/s

3. Calculate one time constant for the following data:
   PIP: 29 cm H_2O
   $P_{plateau}$: 23 cm H_2O
   V_T: 600 cc
   PEEP: 5 cm H_2O
   Inspiratory flow rate: 45 L/min
   a. 0.017 second
   b. 0.021 second
   c. 0.21 second
   d. 0.27 second

4. The cause of a mechanically ventilated patient's PIP increasing from 20 to 40 cm H_2O while the static compliance remains relatively unchanged is which of the following?
   a. Removed mucous plugs
   b. Increased R_{aw}
   c. Tension pneumothorax
   d. Decreased elastance

5. An increase in PIP and $P_{plateau}$ with a stable P_{TA} may be caused by which of the following?
   a. Acute Respiratory Distress Syndrome
   b. Acute asthma exacerbation
   c. Retained secretions in the airways
   d. An endotracheal tube that is too small

6. Which of the following will occur when a patient's lung-thoracic compliance improves?
   1. $P_{plateau}$ decreases
   2. PIP decreases
   3. $P_{plateau}$ increases
   4. P_{TA} increases
   a. 1 and 2 only
   b. 1 and 4 only
   c. 2 and 3 only
   d. 3 and 4 only

7. Over the course of several hours, a respiratory therapist has detected an increase in P_{TA} of a mechanically ventilated patient. The patient's $P_{plateau}$ has remained stable. Which of the following may be the cause of this increase?
   a. Improving lung-thoracic compliance
   b. Acute Respiratory Distress Syndrome
   c. Fluid buildup in the peritoneal cavity
   d. Increase of airway secretions

8. A patient's P_{TA} is rising, while the $P_{plateau}$ is constant. Which of the following should be done to correct this problem?
   1. Administer a bronchodilator
   2. Place a large-bore needle in the third intercostal space
   3. Measure auto-PEEP
   4. Suction airway secretions
   a. 2 only
   b. 3 and 4 only
   c. 1 and 4 only
   d. 1 and 3 only

9. Calculate the static compliance for a patient who is being mechanically ventilated and has an exhaled V_T of 825 mL, $P_{plateau}$ of 47 cm H_2O, and PEEP of 8 cm H_2O.
   a. 15 mL/cm H_2O
   b. 18 mL/cm H_2O
   c. 21 mL/cm H_2O
   d. 47 mL/cm H_2O

10. Which of the following situations will demonstrate the highest airway resistance?
   a. PIP is 65 cm H_2O, $P_{plateau}$ is 55 cm H_2O, flow rate is 60 L/min
   b. PIP is 52 cm H_2O, $P_{plateau}$ is 18 cm H_2O, flow rate is 45 L/min
   c. PIP is 45 cm H_2O, $P_{plateau}$ is 30 cm H_2O, flow rate is 50 L/min
   d. PIP is 30 cm H_2O, $P_{plateau}$ is 10 cm H_2O, flow rate is 40 L/min

Chapter **1** Basic Terms and Concepts of Mechanical Ventilation

HELPFUL INTERNET SITES

- Johns Hopkins School of Medicine's Interactive Respiratory Physiology: Air Flow
  http://oac.med.jhmi.edu/res_phys/Encyclopedia/AirFlow/AirFlow.html
- Johns Hopkins School of Medicine's Interactive Respiratory Physiology: Airway Resistance
  http://oac.med.jhmi.edu/res_phys/Encyclopedia/AirwayResistance/AirwayResistance.html
- Johns Hopkins School of Medicine's Interactive Respiratory Physiology: Alveolar Pressure
  http://oac.med.jhmi.edu/res_phys/Encyclopedia/AlveolarPressure/AlveolarPressure.html
- Johns Hopkins School of Medicine's Interactive Respiratory Physiology: Chest Wall
  http://oac.med.jhmi.edu/res_phys/Encyclopedia/ChestWall/ChestWall.html
- Johns Hopkins School of Medicine's Interactive Respiratory Physiology: Compliance
  http://oac.med.jhmi.edu/res_phys/Encyclopedia/Compliance/Compliance.html
- Simulations in Physiology: The Respiratory System by H.I. Modell and T.W. Modell (free downloadable software)

2 How Ventilators Work

LEARNING OBJECTIVES

On completion of this chapter the reader will be able to do the following:

1. List the basic types of power sources used for mechanical ventilators.
2. Give examples of ventilators that use an electrical power source and a pneumatic power source.
3. Explain the difference in function between positive and negative pressure ventilators.
4. Distinguish between a closed-loop and an open-loop system.
5. Define *user interface*.
6. Describe a ventilator's internal and external pneumatic circuits.
7. Discuss the difference between a single-circuit and a double-circuit ventilator.
8. Identify the components of an external circuit (patient circuit).
9. Explain the function of an externally mounted exhalation valve.
10. Compare the functions of the three different types of volume displacement drive mechanisms.
11. Describe the function of the proportional solenoid valve.

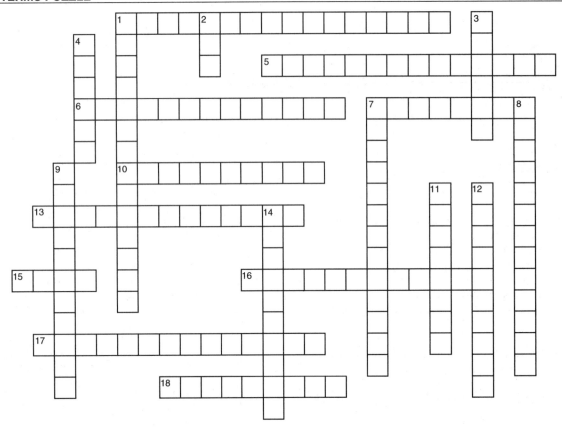

Across

1 A pathway of tubes within the ventilator is an internal _____ (two words)
5 Single chip made of integrated circuits
6 Another name for the control panel (two words)
7 Pneumatic valve that uses an electromagnetic field and is controlled by a microprocessor
10 Device for which the internal volume can be changed
13 What is inside the black box?
15 Type of controller
16 Stepper motor that controls a hinged clamp device (two words)
17 Mechanical device that causes gas to flow to the patient (two words)
18 Uses 50 psi as a power source

Down

1 Connects to the patient (two words)
2 Ventilator mode where the clinician sets a minimum minute ventilation (abbreviation)
3 Mechanism to change internal volume
4 Type of controller
7 From ventilator directly to patient type ventilator (two words)
8 This type of ventilator has two internal pneumatic circuits (two words)
9 Type of valve that controls gas flow (two words)
11 Unintelligent system (two words)
12 Intelligent system (two words)
14 Uses AC or DC as a power source

CHAPTER REVIEW QUESTIONS

1. Name the two types of power sources used by ventilators that provide energy to perform the work of ventilating the patient.

    a. _____

    b. _____

2. What specific power source does each of the following ventilators use?

    Bird Mark 7 _____

    Lifecare PLV-102 _____

    Servo-i _____

    LTV 800, 900, and 1000 _____

    Bio-Med MVP-10 _____

3. Describe an open-loop system.

    _____

    _____

4. Describe a closed-loop system.

    _____

    _____

5. Explain the difference in how gas flows into the lung with positive- versus negative-pressure ventilators.

    _____

    _____

    _____

    _____

6. The position on the ventilator where the clinician inputs and monitors ventilator parameters is known as the _____.

7. List five common components that can be set by the clinician using knobs or touch pads located on the user interface of the ventilator.

    a. _____

    b. _____

    c. _____

    d. _____

    e. _____

8. From your answer to Question 7, what four ventilatory variables do these controls ultimately regulate?

    a. _____

    b. _____

    c. _____

    d. _____

9. Inside a ventilator, gas flow passes through what type of circuit?

    _____

10. After exiting the ventilator, gas flow passes through the _____ on its way to the patient.

11. The gas flow from the ventilator's power source goes directly to the patient. This is known as what type of internal pneumatic circuit?

    _____

12. Describe the difference between single- and double-circuit ventilators. Which is more common in Intensive Care Unit (ICU) ventilators today?

    _____

13. List the four basic elements of a patient circuit.

    a. _____

    b. _____

    c. _____

    d. _____

14. Identify the labeled parts of the ventilator circuit shown in Figure 2-1.

    a. _____

    b. _____

    c. _____

    d. _____

15. Explain how an external exhalation valve operates.

_____

_____

_____

_____

16. In most current ICU ventilators, where are most exhalation valves located?

_____

17. What is the drive mechanism?

_____

18. Name two types of flow-control valves available on current ventilators.

a. _____

b. _____

19. Describe how each of the flow-control valves operates.

_____

_____

_____

_____

_____

_____

20. The internal hardware that converts electrical or pneumatic energy to a system that provides a breath

to a patient is called the _____

21. Name four types of compressors that are used in ventilators.

a. _____

b. _____

c. _____

d. _____

22. Describe how a spring-loaded bellows functions.

_____

_____

_____

23. Describe how a linear drive piston functions.

_____

_____

_____

24. Describe how a rotary drive piston functions.

_____

_____

_____

_____

25. The ICU ventilators used today have what type of internal functions?

_____

_____

CRITICAL THINKING QUESTIONS

1. If the exhalation valve fails to close, what happens to the inspiratory gas flow?

_____

_____

2. What type of ventilator could be used during a magnetic resonance imaging procedure?

_____

CASE STUDIES

Case Study 1

A patient receiving mechanical ventilation needs to be transported to another medical center for treatment. What type of power source would be appropriate for use during patient transport?

_____

_____

Case Study 2

While being mechanically ventilated in a mode that allows spontaneous breathing, a patient becomes apneic. The ventilator automatically alarms and switches to full ventilatory support. Is this an open- or closed-loop system? Explain.

_____

_____

_____

NBRC-STYLE QUESTIONS

1. The power used by a mechanical ventilator to perform the work of ventilating the patient is known as which of the following?
   a. Force
   b. Pressure
   c. Input power
   d. Output power

2. Which of the following statement(s) is (are) true concerning combined power ventilators?
   1. They must have an electrical power source and two 50-psi gas sources.
   2. They often have RAM and ROM for data and preprogrammed modes.
   3. The electrical power provides the energy to deliver the breath.
   4. The pneumatic power controls the internal function of the machine.
   a. 2 only
   b. 1 and 3 only
   c. 3 and 4 only
   d. 1, 2, and 4 only

3. The internal circuit of a ventilator has the gas go directly from its power source to the patient. This is known as which of the following?
   a. External circuit
   b. Internal circuit
   c. Single circuit
   d. Double circuit

4. One of the functions of the exhalation valve is to do which of the following?
   a. Regulate pressure
   b. Ensure adequate humidification
   c. Ensure gas delivery on inspiration
   d. Determine the patient's tidal volume

5. A closed-loop system is used to guarantee a minute ventilation to a patient. The minute ventilation delivered to the patient differs significantly from the set volume. The ventilator will do which of the following?
   a. Alarm and shut off
   b. Switch to 100% oxygen
   c. Deliver the set minute ventilation
   d. Alter the delivered volume

6. The mechanical device that causes gas to flow to the patient is known as which of the following?
   a. Drive mechanism
   b. Power transmission
   c. Exhalation valve
   d. Solenoid valve

7. Volume displacement devices include which of the following?
   1. Pistons
   2. Stepper motors
   3. Concertina bags
   4. Proportional solenoids
   a. 1 and 4 only
   b. 1 and 3 only
   c. 2 and 3 only
   d. 2 and 4 only

8. The flow-control valve that uses an electromagnetic field is which of the following?
   a. Digital valve
   b. Stepper motor
   c. Solenoid valve
   d. Rotating blade

9. Currently, which type of ventilator is most commonly used in ICU?
   a. Fluidic ventilator
   b. Electrically powered ventilator
   c. Pneumatically powered ventilator
   d. Microprocessor controlled ventilator

10. The volume displacement device that creates a sinusoidal flow wave pattern during inspiration is which of the following?
    a. Spring-loaded bellows
    b. Linear drive piston
    c. Rotary drive piston
    d. Concertina bag

HELPFUL INTERNET SITES

- Critical Care Medicine Tutorials: Mechanical Ventilation Medley of Modes
  http://www.ccmtutorials.com/rs/mv/page4.htm
- J.X. Brunner, "History and principles of closed-loop control applied to mechanical ventilation"
  http://alumni.cs.ucr.edu/~kstephen/ventilator/Brunner_2002.pdf

3 How a Breath Is Delivered

LEARNING OBJECTIVES

On completion of this chapter the reader will be able to do the following:

1. Write the equation for motion and define each term in the equation.
2. Give two other names for pressure ventilation and volume ventilation.
3. Compare pressure, volume, and flow delivery in either volume-controlled breaths or pressure-controlled breaths.
4. Name the two most common patient-trigger variables.
5. Identify the patient-trigger variable that requires the least work of breathing for a patient receiving mechanical ventilation.
6. Explain the effect on the volume delivered and the inspiratory time if a ventilator reaches the set maximum pressure limit during volume ventilation.
7. Describe the pressure–time and flow–time waveforms that occur with pressure-support ventilation.
8. Recognize the effects of a critical leak (e.g., a patient disconnect) on pressure readings and volume measurements.
9. Define *inflation hold* and describe its effects on inspiratory time.
10. Give an example of a current ventilator that provides negative pressure during part of the expiratory phase.
11. From a clinical example of ventilator waveforms, identify the triggering, limiting, and cycling mechanisms.
12. Based on the description of a pressure–time curve, identify a clinical situation in which expiratory resistance is increased.
13. Compare the terms *time cycling*, *volume cycling*, and *flow cycling* as they might be applied to a microprocessor-controlled ventilator in a volume-controlled mode using a set machine rate and flow.
14. Define the following terms, and explain how these factors affect a breath: *expiratory retard*, *positive end-expiratory pressure* (PEEP), *continuous positive airway pressure*, and *bilevel positive airway pressure*.

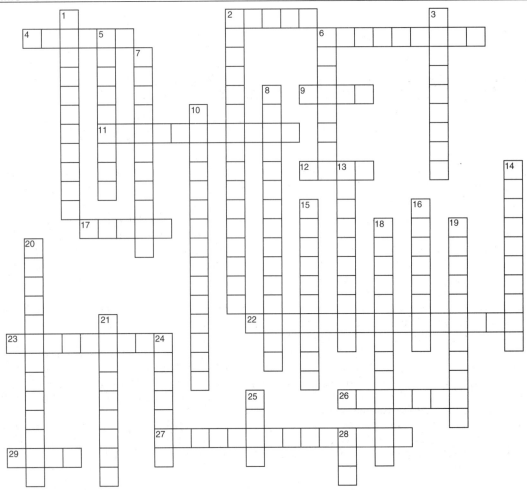

Across

2 Variable that ends inspiration
4 Specific amount that begins inspiration
6 Gas law that governs tubing compressibility (two words)
9 Applying positive pressure during expiration during mechanical ventilation (abbreviation)
11 The ventilator begins inspiration (two words)
12 Applying negative pressure during expiration (abbreviation)
17 Maximum value a variable can attain
22 Primary variable the ventilator uses to cause inspiration (two words)
23 Gas speed reaches a maximum amount (two words)
26 Pressure read during an inspiratory pause
27 Maneuver performed to measure auto-PEEP (two words)
29 A baseline pressure at zero (abbreviation)

Down

1 Gas speed begins inspiration (two words)
2 The way a ventilator marks the end of inspiration (two words)
3 Most common mechanism for ending inspiration in the pressure support mode (two words)
5 A breath initiated by the ventilator is a _____ breath.
6 Pressure level from which a ventilator breath begins
7 Maxed out at an amount (two words)
8 Pressure target ventilator mode where the patient breathes spontaneously (two words)
10 Ventilator mode where the set limit is pressure (two words)
13 Breathing out
14 The patient is making no effort—ventilation is being _____ by the ventilator.
15 Breathing in
16 Variable that begins inspiration
18 Variable controlling a certain phase of a breath (two words)
19 A breath controlled by the patient
20 A breath begun by the operator (two words)
21 The ventilator ends inspiration (two words)
24 Variable that begins inspiration
25 Application of pressures above ambient throughout inspiration and expiration to a spontaneously breathing patient (abbreviation)
28 Type of ventilation that assists both inspiration and expiration (abbreviation)

CHAPTER REVIEW QUESTIONS

1. The equation for motion is

   _____

2. List two ways the energy required to produce motion can be achieved.

   a. _____

   b. _____

3. Explain all of the elements of the equation for motion.

   _____

   _____

   _____

   _____

4. List two factors that determine the way the inspiratory volume is delivered.

   a. _____

   b. _____

5. List two synonyms for pressure-controlled ventilation.

   a. _____

   b. _____

6. List two synonyms for volume-controlled ventilation.

   a. _____

   b. _____

7. List four variables that a ventilator can control during inspiration.

   a. _____

   b. _____

   c. _____

   d. _____

8. The primary variable that a ventilator adjusts to produce inspiration is called _____.

9. During pressure-controlled breaths, the compliance and resistance of a patient's lungs change. What happens to volume and flow?

   _____

   _____

10. If during volume-controlled breaths the patient's lung compliance decreases, what will happen to the peak inspiratory pressure (PIP)?

    _____

    _____

11. Explain your answer to Question 10.

    _____

    _____

12. Both pressure and volume waveforms can be affected by changes in lung characteristics while what type of control variable is being used?

    _____

13. What two types of ventilators deliver a time-controlled breath?

    a. _____

    b. _____

14. Describe the relationship between flow and volume in the form of a formula.

    _____

15. List the three places where ventilators measure pressure.

    a. _____

    b. _____

    c. _____

16. The pressure, volume, and flow waveforms can take one of four shapes. List each below.

    a. _____

    b. _____

    c. _____

    d. _____

17. List the phase variables of a breath.

    a. _____

    b. _____

    c. _____

    d. _____

18. The phase variable that begins inspiration is known as the _____

19. Patient triggering is based on _____, _____, or _____ changes.

20. The ventilator initiates a breath after a set time. What phase variable is this describing? _____

21. Describe the limit variable.

_____

22. Describe the cycle variable. _____

23. Describe the baseline variable. _____

24. Explain auto-triggering.

_____

_____

25. At which pressure would it be easier for a patient to initiate a breath? -1 cm H_2O or -3 cm H_2O. At which flow would it be easier for a patient to initiate a breath? 2 L/min or 4 L/min. (Circle the correct answers.)

26. If the flow sensitivity is set at 2 L/min and the baseline flow is 6 L/min, at what flow will the ventilator be triggered to give a breath? _____

27. When set properly by the clinician, which triggering method has been shown to require less work of breathing for the patient? _____

28. Describe volume triggering.

_____

_____

Questions 29 through 32 refer to Figure 3-1.

29. What is the control variable? _____

30. What is the expiratory time? _____

31. What is the inspiratory time? _____

32. What is the baseline? _____

Questions 33 through 36 refer to Figure 3-2

33. What type of trigger does wave A have?

_____

34. What type of trigger does wave B have?

_____

35. What type of trigger does wave C have?

_____

36. What is the baseline? _____

37. The maximum value that a variable can attain is known as a _____.

Questions 38 through 42: Classify the following breaths as mandatory, assisted, or spontaneous.

38. Pressure-triggered, pressure-limited, time-cycled:

_____

39. Flow-triggered, volume-limited, time-cycled:

_____

40. Time-triggered, pressure-limited, time-cycled:

_____

41. Flow-triggered, patient-cycled:

_____

42. Pressure-triggered, flow-limited, volume-limited, volume-cycled:

_____

43. Do limits cycle a breath? _____

44. When the set high-pressure limit is reached during inspiration, what happens (if using the Covidien PB 840)?

_____

_____

45. List three names ventilator manufacturers use for the maximum pressure-control function.

a. _____

b. _____

c. _____

46. Typically, how does the clinician determine the maximum safety pressure?

_____

47. What is the internal maximum safety pressure used by most ventilator manufacturers?

_____

48. How do most Intensive Care Unit (ICU) ventilators achieve volume cycling?

_____

_____

49. What is the tubing compressibility factor for most adult ventilator circuits?

_____

50. How much volume will be lost in the patient circuit when the tubing compressibility is 2.5 mL/cm H_2O, the set volume is 500 mL, 0 PEEP, and the PIP is 25 cm H_2O?

_____

51. Give two reasons why exhaled tidal volume (V_T) may not equal the set V_T when a breath is volume cycled.

a. _____

b. _____

52. A large leak is detected in the ventilator system during pressure-support ventilation. How will the ventilator end inspiration?

_____

53. The ventilator cycles to expiration when the patient's exhaled gas flow drops to a certain percentage of the peak inspiratory flow rate. This describes what type of end to inspiration?

_____

54. Give a clinical scenario where a pressure-cycled ventilator could be used.

_____

_____

55. How does flow cycling occur during pressure-support ventilation?

_____

_____

_____

56. What flow is required to deliver 600 mL in 1 second with a constant gas flow?

_____

_____

57. What happens to inspiratory and expiratory times during an inflation hold?

_____

58. List three terms also used to describe an inflation hold.

a. _____

b. _____

c. _____

59. Air trapping can occur following an inflation hold if

_____

60. Define the expiratory phase.

_____

61. The pressure level from which a ventilator breath begins is called the _____.

62. The addition of a positive pressure to exhalation during mechanical ventilation is called

_____.

63. What type of ventilator assists both inspiration and expiration by pushing air into the lungs and pulling it back out at extremely high frequencies?

_____

64. A patient who is intubated and receiving mechanical ventilation is allowed to exhale. The ventilator then closes both expiratory and inspiratory valves.

This maneuver is known as _____ and

measures the amount of _____

65. Increased resistance to exhalation may be caused by what devices?

_____

66. The application of pressures above ambient throughout inspiration and expiration to improve oxygenation in a spontaneously breathing patient is

referred to as _____.

67. What are the two pressure sets during bilevel positive pressure ventilation (NIV)?

a. _____

b. _____

CRITICAL THINKING QUESTIONS

Questions 1 through 6 refer to Figure 3-3, which shows a pressure–time curve and flow–time curve.

1. What is the limit mechanism for these breaths?

_____

2. Name the three possible modes that these graphs represent.

a. _____

b. _____

c. _____

3. What is the trigger mechanism for the breaths shown?

_____

4. What is the cycling mechanism for the breaths shown?

_____

5. What is the inspiratory time? _____

6. What is the expiratory time? _____

Questions 7 through 10 refer to Figure 3-4.

7. What is the trigger variable for waveform *A*?

_____

8. What is the trigger variable for waveform *B*?

_____

9. The transairway pressure is _____.

10. What is the baseline? _____

CASE STUDIES

Case Study 1

You are a respiratory therapist assigned to the ICU of a local hospital and have been called to assess a patient who may require mechanical ventilation. Physical examination reveals a respiratory rate of 25, blood pressure 145/90, pulse 115, and breath sounds are bilaterally decreased, especially in the bases. The arterial blood gas reveals:
pH 7.44
P_aCO_2 36 mm Hg
P_aO_2 42 mm Hg
S_aO_2 70%
HCO_3^- 22 mEq/L
Device: a nonrebreather mask at 10 L/min
The patient's maximal inspiratory pressure is -75 cm H_2O, VC is 70 mL/kg, and V_T is 7 mL/kg.

1. Explain the primary area of concern for this patient.

_____

_____

_____

2. What is the most appropriate type of ventilatory support for this patient at this time?

_____

_____

The following day you return to the ICU and find this patient is receiving mechanical ventilation. Figure 3-5 shows the graphic display.

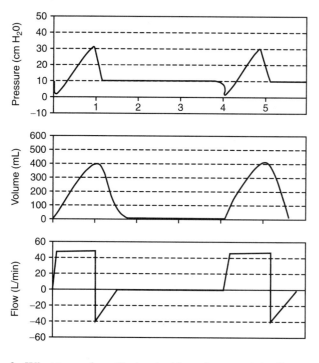

3. What type of ventilation is this patient receiving?

_____

4. What is(are) the limiting variable(s)?

_____

5. What trigger variable is being used at this time?

_____

In addition, you note that the patient is diaphoretic and is using accessory muscles while assisting.

6. Do any of the graphic displays give clues to the source of this patient's problem? If so, which one(s)?

_____

7. What is likely the source of this patient's problem?

_____

_____

_____

8. To alleviate this problem, what should you do?

_____

_____

_____

Case Study 2

A postoperative patient is being placed on a mechanical ventilator in volume-controlled ventilation.

1. What parameters need to be set by the respiratory therapist?

_____

_____

2. During mechanical ventilation, the patient's PIP is reaching 28 cm H_2O. At what level should the maximum safety pressure be set?

_____

3. What is the purpose of the maximum safety pressure?

_____

_____

While performing a patient-ventilator assessment, the respiratory therapist notices that although a V_T of 500 mL is set, only an exhaled V_T of 400 mL is being measured, and the maximum safety pressure is reached during each breath.

4. What is the most likely cause for the difference between set and exhaled V_T? Explain your answer.

_____

_____

_____

5. If the maximum safety pressure was not reached on each breath and the exhaled volume was 100 mL less than the set V_T, what could be the possible causes?

_____

_____

NBRC-STYLE QUESTIONS

1. A breath that is triggered, limited, and cycled by the mechanical ventilator is which of the following?
   a. Assisted
   b. Mandatory
   c. Spontaneous
   d. Synchronized

2. A breath that is triggered, controlled, and ended by the patient is which of the following?
   a. Assisted
   b. Controlled
   c. Spontaneous
   d. Synchronized

Chapter **3** **How a Breath Is Delivered**

3. A breath that is patient triggered, ventilator controlled, and cycled is which of the following?
   a. Assisted
   b. Controlled
   c. Spontaneous
   d. Pressure supported

4. During pressure-controlled ventilation, the patient's airway resistance (R_{aw}) increases. This will cause which of the following to occur?
   a. The peak pressure will increase.
   b. The peak pressure will decrease.
   c. The delivered V_T will increase.
   d. The delivered V_T will decrease.

5. During volume-controlled ventilation the patient's lung compliance improves. This will cause which of the following to occur?
   a. The peak pressure will increase.
   b. The peak pressure will decrease.
   c. The delivered V_T will increase.
   d. The delivered V_T will decrease.

6. During volume-controlled ventilation, which waveform remains unchanged with changes in the patient's lung characteristics?
   1. Volume–time curve
   2. Pressure–time curve
   3. Flow–time curve
   a. 1 only
   b. 2 only
   c. 1 and 3 only
   d. 2 and 3 only

7. When both pressure and volume waveforms are affected by changes in lung characteristics, which of following variables is being controlled?
   a. Time
   b. Flow
   c. Volume
   d. Pressure

8. A high-frequency oscillator controls which of the following variables?
   a. Flow
   b. Time
   c. Volume
   d. Pressure

9. When the ventilator is time triggering and the rate is set at 20 breaths/min, the time interval between breaths is which of the following?
   a. 2 seconds
   b. 3 seconds
   c. 4 seconds
   d. 5 seconds

10. During flow triggering the base flow is set at 5 L/min and the ventilator triggers when it senses 3 L/min returning to its flow measuring device. The flow sensitivity setting is which of the following?
    a. 2 L/min
    b. 3 L/min
    c. 5 L/min
    d. 8 L/min

11. During pressure-support ventilation the patient triggers the ventilator, the set pressure is reached, and the ventilator cycles at 5 seconds. What is the cause of this time cycle?
    a. A leak in the system.
    b. This is the normal setting.
    c. Increased lung compliance.
    d. Change in R_{aw}.

12. The most common cycling mechanism used for pressure-support ventilation is which of the following?
    a. Time
    b. Flow
    c. Volume
    d. Pressure

13. The maneuver used to measure plateau pressure is which of the following?
    a. Flow limiting
    b. Expiratory hold
    c. Inspiratory hold
    d. Pressure limiting

14. What is the transrespiratory pressure if the ventilator is set at a volume of 500 mL with a flow of 60 L/min and the patient's lung compliance is 0.75 L/cm H_2O and R_{aw} is 6 cm H_2O/L/s?
    a. 0.12 cm H_2O
    b. 4.5 cm H_2O
    c. 6.7 cm H_2O
    d. 7.5 cm H_2O

15. What flow is needed to deliver 850 mL of volume to a patient in 0.75 second with a constant gas flow?
    a. 53 L/min
    b. 60 L/min
    c. 68 L/min
    d. 75 L/min

HELPFUL INTERNET SITES

- Welcome to the WorldWide Anaesthetist, "New Approaches to Mechanical Ventilation" http://www.anaesthetist.com/anaes/vent/Findex.htm#index.htm
- Hamilton Medical, HAMILTON G5 Online Simulation http://www.hamilton-medical.com/Online-simulation.683.0.html

4 Establishing the Need for Mechanical Ventilation

LEARNING OBJECTIVES

Upon completion of this chapter the reader will be able to do the following:

1. Differentiate between acute respiratory failure (ARF) and respiratory distress.
2. Identify goals and objectives of mechanical ventilation.
3. List the respiratory, cardiovascular, and neurological findings in mild, moderate, and severe hypercapnia.
4. Describe three categories of disorders that may lead to respiratory insufficiency or acute respiratory failure.
5. Compare normal values for the vital capacity, maximum inspiratory force, peak expiratory pressure, forced expiratory volume in 1 second (FEV_1), peak expiratory flow rate, physiological dead space/tidal volume (V_D/V_T) ratio, alveolar–arterial oxygen pressure difference ($P[A - a]O_2$), and arterial to alveolar partial pressure of oxygen (P_aO_2/P_AO_2) ratio with abnormal values that indicate the need for ventilatory support.
6. Evaluate patient cases and recommend appropriate respiratory therapy interventions including oxygen therapy, bronchodilator therapy, continuous positive airway pressure (CPAP), noninvasive positive-pressure ventilation (NIV), and positive pressure invasive ventilation.
7. Discuss circumstances in which mechanical ventilation would be inappropriate even though the patient meets the standard criteria.

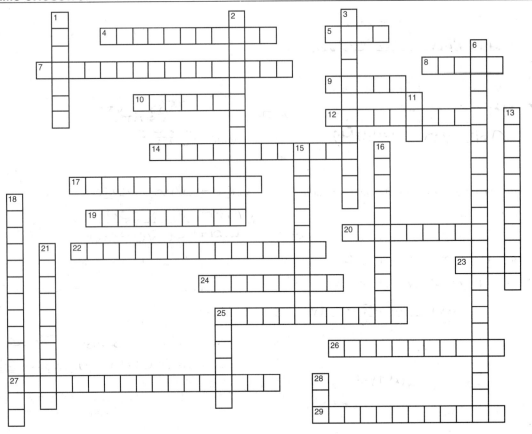

Across

4 Pertaining to the space between the ribs
5 An indicator of airway obstruction (abbreviation)
7 Type of neuromuscular disease that causes descending paralysis
8 Condition in which perfusion of vital organs is inadequate to meet their metabolic needs
9 Breathing that has irregular periods of apnea alternating with periods of deep breathing
10 Type of respiratory failure also referred to as *lung failure*
12 Sleepiness
14 Type of neuromuscular disease that causes descending paralysis
17 Respiratory failure referred to as *pump failure*
19 Type of hypoxemia that is resistant to treatment
20 Rapid breathing
22 Controversial treatment for a closed head wound
23 State of unconsciousness
24 State of lethargy and immobility with diminished responsiveness to stimulation
25 Above the sternum
26 Normal respiratory balance
27 Latin for acute, severe asthma (two words)
29 An abnormal breathing pattern characterized by alternating progressive hypopnea and hypoventilation ending in brief apnea (two words)

Down

1 Pus in the pleural space
2 Measurement used to assess respiratory muscle strength (two words)
3 Device used to measure volumes at the bedside
6 Absent or inadequate respiratory activity (three words)
11 Condition characterized by alveolar flooding caused by an acute insult (abbreviation)
13 Breathing pattern characterized by abnormal movement of the thorax and abdomen
15 Breathing pattern in which the rib cage and abdomen do not move outward together
16 Early indicator of hypoxemia
18 Abnormal anteroposterior and lateral curvature of the spine
21 Blood in the pleural space
25 Toxic condition arising from infection
28 When increasing lung volume this increases (abbreviation)

Chapter **4 Establishing the Need for Mechanical Ventilation**

CHAPTER REVIEW QUESTIONS

1. What is the primary purpose of ventilation?

   To Maintain homeostasis

2. List and explain the components of the three basic physiological objectives of mechanical ventilation?

   Support of (see pg 44).
   a. manipulate Pulmonary gas exchange
   b. Increase lung volume
   c. Reduce the work of breathing

3. List eight clinical objectives of mechanical ventilation.

   Reverse
   a. cute respiratory failure
   b. Reverse respiratory distress
   c. Reverse hypoxemia
   Prevent
   d. or reverse atelectasis & maintain FRC.
   e. Reverse respiratory Muscle fatigue
   f. Permit Sedation or Paralysis (or both)
   Reduce systemic or Myocardial Oxygen Consumption
   g.
   Minimize associated complications & reduce
   h.
   mortality.

4. List 10 physical signs of respiratory distress.

   a. Tachypnea
   b. Nasal flaring
   c. diaphoresis
   d. accessory Muscle use
   retractions of Suprasternal, Supraclavicular +
   e. intercostal site
   Paradoxical, or thorax + abdomen.
   f.
   g. Abnormal breath Sounds
   h. tachycardia
   i. arrhythmia
   j. hypotension.

5. When respiratory activity is inadequate to maintain oxygen uptake and carbon dioxide clearance, it is referred to as Acute respiratory Failure (ARF).

6. Clinically, what arterial blood gas (ABG) measurements indicate ARF? A PaO2 below
   the predicted normal range for the Patient
   age under ambient conditions.
   a.
   a PaCo2 greater than 50mg & rising
   b.
   c. a falling PH of 7.25 or lower.

7. List and define the two forms of acute respiratory failure and give examples of each. (see pg 45)

   a. Acute life-threatening
   b. Acute hypercapnic respiratory failure.

8. Basic treatment for hypoxemic respiratory failure includes Oxygen and PEEP possibly in combination with CPAP

9. What does the ventilatory pump consist of?
   Respiratory Muscles, thoracic Cage, nerves & nerve Centers that Control ventilation.

10. List five disorders that reduce the drive to breathe.

    a. Brain or brainstem lesions
    b. depressant drugs
    c. hypothyroidism
    d. central sleep apnea
    e. inappropriate oxygen therapy.

11. List five disorders associated with neuromuscular function that can cause hypoventilation and possible respiratory failure.

    a. Myasthenia gravis
    b. Guillain-Barre Syndrome
    c. Poliomyelitis
    d. Muscular dystrophy
    e. amyotrophic lateral sclerosis.

12. What chest wall deformities result in increased work of breathing? Flail Chest, rib fracture, Kyphoscoliosis, & obesity

13. What pulmonary diseases cause increased airway resistance and result in increased work of breathing?
    Asthma, emphysema, Chronic bronchitis, Croup, acute epiglottis and acute bronchitis

14. What should be included in an initial rapid assessment of a patient with possible respiratory failure? Level of consciousness, Presence of Cyanosis & or diaphoresis, respiratory rate, heart rate, blood pressure, SpO2 & temperature

(27)

15. Fill in the following chart as it relates to the conditions seen with hypoxemia and hypercapnia.

See PG 45   4°2

HYPOXEMIA

	Mild to Moderate	Severe
Respiratory findings	Tachypnea Dyspnea, Pallor	Tachypnea Dyspnea, Cyanosis
Cardiovascular findings	Tachycardia Hypertension	Tachycardia
Neurologic findings	Restlesseness Disorientat	Confusion Blurred vision.

HYPERCAPNIA

	Mild to Moderate	Severe
Respiratory findings	Tachycardia Dyspnea	Tachypnea
Cardiovascular findings	Tachycardia Hypertension	Tachycardia
Neurologic findings	Headaches Drowsiness	Hallucinations
Signs	Sweating	

16. What three elements are required to successfully treat a patient in acute or impending respiratory failure?

Use of Supplemental Oxygen therapy Maintenance of Pt airway Continuous monitoring of oxygenation ventilatory status Pulse oximetry + ABGS

17. Patients with central nervous system dysfunctions may exhibit what two breathing patterns?

a. *Cheyne-Stokes breathing*

b. *Biot's breathing*

18. How often should a patient with a neuromuscular disorder and respiratory fatigue be monitored for changes in respiratory status?

Every 2-4 hours

19. What two measurements should be used to monitor a patient with a neuromuscular disorder and respiratory fatigue to test for muscle strength? What are their critical values?

a. *Vital Capacity equal less than 10-15 ML*

b. *a maximum inspiratory pressure between 0 and -20 cm H2O,*

20. What limits tolerance to an increased work of breathing?

Respiratory muscle fatigue.

21. List three signs of increased work of breathing.

a. *Tachypnea*

b. *increased depth of respiration*

c. *paradoxical breathing*

22. What is a normal maximum inspiratory pressure (MIP)?

-50 to -100 cm H2O

23. What is another name for MIP? *Negative inspiratory force (NIF).*

24. MIP measurement stops when the lowest negative value is reached, which can take up to _____*20*_____ seconds.

25. What is the normal range for vital capacity?

65 - 75 mL/kg

26. ARF is most likely present when minute ventilation exceeds

10L/min

27. What pulmonary function parameter can be used at the bedside to identify increased airway resistance? What measurement is considered critical?

FEV_1, less than 10 mL/kg

28. An indicator of adequate airway patency and airway resistance is *Peak expiratory Flow rate*. What measurement is considered critical? *less than 75-100 L/min*

29. Adequate ventilation can be determined by looking at what ABG value? *$PaCO_2$*

30. The normal VD/VT range is between *0.3, 0/4* and *0.4* at normal tidal volumes. The critical value for this measurement is *greater than 0.6*

31. List three common causes of increased dead space ventilation.

a. *Pulmonary thromboemboli*

b. *Pulmonary vascular injury*

c. *regional hypoperfusion.*

32. Complete the following table for oxygen status assessment.

Measurement	Normal Range	Critical Value
$P(A - a)O_2$	2-30 mm room air	Greater than 450, Supplement
P_aO_2/P_AO_2	0.75 0.195	Less than 0.15
P_aO_2/F_IO_2	475	Less than 200

33. A patient with congestive heart failure is receiving NIV. The patient is not responding well to this therapy. What action should be taken at this time?

Intubate & mechanically ventilate the patient

34. What are the two key indicators of the severity of acute hypoxemic respiratory failure?

PaO_2 & SpO_2

35. Based on ABG values, list five indications that suggest the need for invasive mechanical ventilation.

(See pg 47 4°2 Table)

Normal
a. 7.35 - 7.45   < 7.25
b. 35-45   > 55 +
c. 0.3 - 0.4   > 0.6
d. 80-100   < 70 (On O_2 7.06)
e. 30 -   > 450 (on O_2)

36. In what type of situation would intubation be contraindicated?

When it is contrary to the pt wishes, medically pointless or futile.

37. List three indications for NIV in an adult.

a. Respiratory rate >25 breaths/mins
b. Severe acidosis (pH 7.25-7.30) & PaCO2 45-60 mmHg
c. Mod to sev dyspnea, muscles, paradoxical breathing pattern,

38. List five absolute contraindications for NIV in an adult.

a. Respiratory arrest
b. Cardiac arrest
c. Non-respiratory organ failure
d. Upper airway obstruction
e. Inability to protect airway or high risk of aspiratory.

39. A 48-year-old woman with a past medical history of congestive heart failure and hypertension is brought to the emergency department (ED) complaining of an acute onset of dyspnea. The patient has frothy pink sputum, pulse is 120 beats/min and irregular, and respirations are 26 breaths/min and labored. Breath sounds reveal bilateral basilar crackles and rhonchi. ABG results: pH 7.31, P_aCO_2 48 mm Hg, P_aO_2 50 mm Hg, S_aO_2 72% on a nonrebreathing mask at 10 L/min. What respiratory therapy modalities should be recommended for this patient?

• bipap   ①
• CPAP app   ②
• Venalator   ③

hypotension =

40. A 79-year-old male with inoperable lung cancer develops acute severe dyspnea. The patient's pulse is 104 beats/min and regular and respirations are 24 breaths/min with accessory muscles being used. Breath sounds are decreased bilaterally in the bases. What treatment should the respiratory therapist recommend for this patient?

• O_2 therapy
• Bronchodilator threatmat

41. A 51-year-old woman presented to the ED complaining of shortness of breath and chest tightness for 2 days. Physical exam reveals pulse 122 beats/min and respirations 35 breaths/min with accessory muscle use. Breath sounds reveal bilateral inspiratory and expiratory wheezing with diminished breath sounds in the bases. The patient is alert and oriented but extremely anxious. ABGs reveal pH 7.22, P_aCO_2 55 mm Hg, and P_aO_2 51 mm Hg on room air. What course of treatment is most appropriate for this patient?

• Respitory, acidois with mild hypoxiema. → O_2 therapy.
• ↓ Bronchodilator treatmat
• Albuterol

exacerbation - worsning

42. A 65-year-old male was admitted this morning with an exacerbation of chronic obstructive pulmonary disease (COPD). Physical exam reveals pulse 107 beats/min and regular, respirations 24 breaths/min and slightly labored, oral temperature 38.5° C, and BP 141/90 mm Hg. Breath sounds are much decreased, especially in the bases. ABG results show pH 7.44, P_aCO_2 33 mm Hg, P_aO_2 52 mm Hg, and HCO_3^- 33 mEq/L. What recommendations should the respiratory therapist make for this patient?

If PaO_2 low = O_2 therapy.
Bronco diolator therapy
_____
_____

43. A 23-year-old male is brought to the ED via ambulance following a bicycle accident in which he suffered head trauma. The patient is unresponsive, pulse is 112 beats/min and regular, respirations are 40 breaths/min and shallow, and breath sounds are decreased throughout. ABG reveals pH 7.21, P_aCO_2 59 mm Hg, and P_aO_2 50 mm Hg on a nasal cannula at 6 L/min. What recommendations should the respiratory therapist make for this patient?

Respitory acidocied, Moderate
hypoxenia.
• intabation
• Ventalation + Oxygen.
_____

44. Calculate the arterial oxygen content for a patient with the following ABG results: pH 7.44, P_aCO_2 44 mm Hg, P_aO_2 59 mm Hg, S_aO_2 91%, F_iO_2 0.21, hemoglobin (Hb) 12 g/dL. Show all work.

$(12 \times 1.34) \times SaO_2 + (PaO_2 \times 0.003)$
$16.08 \times 0.91 + (PaO_2 \times 0.0003)$
$14.6328 + \qquad 0.1829$
$14.63 + 0.18 = 14.81$ VOL%

45. Calculate the arterial oxygen content for a patient with the following ABG results: pH 7.34, P_aCO_2 22 mm Hg, P_aO_2 58 mm Hg, S_aO_2 90%, Hb 8 g/dL. Show all work.

$8 \times 1.34 \times SaO_2 + (PaO_2 \times 0.0003$
$10.72 \times 0.90 = 9.65$
$9.65. \quad + \quad 58 \times .003$
$= 9.82$ VOL%

46. Calculate the arterial oxygen content for a patient with the following ABG results: pH 7.36, P_aCO_2 59 mm Hg, P_aO_2 48 mm Hg, S_aO_2 79%, Hb 17 g/dL. Show all work.

$17 \times 1.34 = 22.78$
$0.79 \times 22.78 = 18. +$
$48 \times .003 = 0.144 + 18 =$
$= 18.14$ VOL%

47. Calculate the P(A − a)O_2 for a patient with the following ABG results: pH 7.31, P_aCO_2 48 mm Hg, P_aO_2 50 mm Hg, S_aO_2 72% on a nonrebreathing mask at 12 L/min. (Assume the nonrebreathing mask is delivering approximately 70% oxygen.) Show all work.

$0.7(760 - 47) = 713$
$713 \times 0.7 = 499.1$
$48 \div 0.8 = 60$
$499 - 60 = 439.$

48. Calculate the arterial/alveolar PO_2 for the patient in Question 47. What does this mean and is this a critical value? $PaO_2 \div PAO_2$
$50 \div 439 = 0.11$
_____

49. Calculate the P_aO_2/F_iO_2 for the patient in Question 47. (Assume the nonrebreathing mask is delivering approximately 70% oxygen.) Is this a critical value?

$50 \cdot 0.7 = 71.43$
_____

50. Calculate the P(A − a)O_2 for the patient with the following ABG results: pH 7.22, P_aCO_2 55 mm Hg, P_aO_2 51 mm Hg on room air. Is this value an indication for mechanical ventilation?

$.21(760 - 47) = 713$
$713 \times .21 = 150 =$
$55 \div 0.8 = 69$
$150 - 69 = 81, 51 = 30.$

51. Calculate the arterial/alveolar PO_2 for the patient in Question 50. Is this a critical value?

$PaO_2 \div PAO_2$
$51 \div 30 = 20.63.$

52. Calculate the P_aO_2/F_IO_2 for the patient in Question 50. Is this a critical value?

_____

_____

_____

_____

CRITICAL THINKING QUESTIONS

1. You are called to the ED to perform a cardiopulmonary assessment of a patient who has just been brought in following a motor vehicle accident. What would be your rapid physical assessment? *Pt - colour*

   Vitals, listen to the lungs.

   Patient Name, Date of Birth

   _____

   _____

2. Following your initial physical assessment of the patient in Question 1, what diagnostic evaluations should be done to assess the need for mechanical ventilation?

   ABG, Chest X-ray, Pulse

   Oxometry.

3. Describe how a patient in respiratory distress might look.

   Pale./Blue, flushed, trypod position,

   leaning forward, using

   neck muscles.

4. Discuss the difference in clinical presentation between a patient needing oxygen therapy only and one who needs mechanical ventilation.

   O2 - Would, Normal PaCO2

   _____

   Mechanical - Ventilation, would have
   low PaO2 & high PaCo2.

CASE STUDIES

Case Study 1

A 35-year-old male, with a history of asthma, was admitted from the ED to the Intensive Care Unit (ICU). The patient is alert, oriented, extremely anxious, sitting up, and leaning on the bedside tray table. Physical exam reveals pulse 142 beats/min, blood pressure (BP) 178/86 mm Hg, oral temperature 37.9° C, and respirations 33 breaths/min and labored. Chest auscultation reveals significantly decreased breath sounds throughout with slight wheezing on exhalation. ABG results on 40% air entrainment mask include the following:
pH 7.33 *↓ acid*
P_aCO_2 44 mm Hg *ok.*
P_aO_2 48 mm Hg *mod - hy*
S_aO_2 79% *↓*
HCO_3^- 22 mEq/L *ok.*
Hb 14.8 g/dL
Peak expiratory flow reading is 70 L/min following three consecutive bronchodilator treatments.

1. What is the most likely cause of the patient's tachycardia?
   hypoxemia + anxious.

   _____

2. Using oxygenation indicators, explain the oxygenation status of this patient. (Assume P_B is 760.)
   Pa O2 ÷ FiO2
   48 ÷ 0.4 = 120.

3. Although this patient's P_aCO_2 is within normal limits, why is it significant in this case?
   Stage 3 of impending
   respiratory failure.

4. What respiratory care treatment should be suggested for this patient?
   ① bronchodilator therapy
   ② up FiO2
   ③ Meds Magnesium Sufate &
   Steroids.
   ④ Ventilatory support, if
   nothing else works.

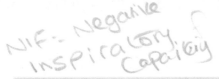
NIF: Negative
Inspiratory
Capacity

Case Study 2

A 46-year-old female was admitted to the ICU a few hours ago with an acute exacerbation of myasthenia gravis. She is alert and oriented, pulse is 102 beats/min and regular, BP is 140/75 mm Hg, oral temperature is 37.4° C, and respirations are 30 breaths/min and very shallow. Breath sounds are decreased throughout. She cannot cough. The patient is complaining of weakness and difficulty swallowing. ABGs on room air reveal pH 7.36, $PaCO_2$ 38 mm Hg, PaO_2 60 mm Hg, SaO_2 90%, HCO_3^- 20 mEq/L, and Hb 12.6 g/dL. Maximum inspiratory pressure is 30 cm H_2O.

1. What is this patient's oxygenation status? Explain your answer. PaO2-60

   Mild, hypoxemia SaO2 Low
   HCO3-Low, PaO2 is 60 it is
   Mild hypoxemia.

2. Evaluate this patient's ventilatory status.

   PH + PaCO2 is normal no
   need to vent.

3. What treatment or monitoring recommendations should be made for this patient? NIF and

   Vital cap, Low flow
   Oxygen as PaO2 is only
   _60._

Case Study 3

A 76-year-old female presents to the ED in severe respiratory failure due to COPD. Her ABG results show pH 7.15, $PaCO_2$ 90 mm Hg, PaO_2 43 mm Hg, HCO_3^- 29 mEq/L, SaO_2 52% on FIO_2 0.4, and CPAP 5 cm H_2O. The patient appears drowsy.

1. What is this patient's oxygenation status? Explain your answer.

   Severe hypoxemic respir
   failure.

2. Evaluate this patient's ventilatory status.

   PH is Low + PaCO2 is
   High pt is in acute
   ventilatory failure.

3. What treatment or monitoring recommendations should be made for this patient?

   Intubation, based on ABG's
   Pt is also drowsy.

NBRC-STYLE QUESTIONS

1. A 43-year-old male was admitted last night with a stab wound to the right anterior thorax. The wound was repaired in surgery. Currently the patient is alert and continuously tries to remove his oxygen mask. He is in the ICU and has a chest tube in his right hemithorax. Vital signs show pulse 120 beats/min, respirations 36 breaths/min and shallow, BP 148/90 mm Hg, and oral temperature 38° C. Breath sounds are decreased over the right base, and chest expansion is decreased over the right side. The patient is not coughing. ABG results reveal pH 7.48, $PaCO_2$ 26 mm Hg, PaO_2 66 mm Hg, SaO_2 94%, HCO_3^- 19 mEq/L, FIO_2 0.55 (via air entrainment mask), and Hb 11.4. Which of the following is the most appropriate action to take at this time?
   a. Increase FIO_2 to 0.5.
   b. Place patient on bilevel positive airway pressure.
   c. Administer albuterol via small volume nebulizer.
   d. Intubate and mechanically ventilate with an FIO_2 of 1.0.

2. Which of the following characterizes hypercapnic respiratory failure?
   1. Lower than normal PaO_2
   2. Alveolar hypoventilation
   3. Higher than normal $PaCO_2$
   4. Increased $PAO_2 - PaO_2$
   a. 1 and 2 only
   b. 1, 2, and 3 only
   c. 2 and 3 only
   d. 2, 3, and 4 only

3. The underlying physiological process leading to pure hypercapnic respiratory failure is which of the following?
   a. Low V/Q ratio
   b. Diffusion impairment
   c. Intrapulmonary shunting
   d. Alveolar hypoventilation

hypercapnic = PaCO2 & alveolar
hypoventilation.
hypoventilation - slow breath not
deep enough.

4. A 65-year-old male presents to the ED complaining of increasing shortness of breath over the past 3 days and appears to be in moderate respiratory distress. He has a 100-pack-year smoking history. Vital signs are heart rate 115 beats/min, respiratory rate 32 breaths/min, BP 170/95 mm Hg, mild expiratory wheezing in his bases, and temperature 100° F oral. His ABG values on nasal cannula 3 L/min are pH 7.30, P_aCO_2 70 mm Hg, P_aO_2 48 mm Hg, S_aO_2 67%, and HCO_3^- 35 mEq/L. The most appropriate treatment at this time is to initiate which of the following?
   a. Bronchodilator therapy
   b. Air entrainment mask at 35%
   c. Intubation and mechanical ventilation
   d. Noninvasive positive pressure ventilation

5. A 55-year-old female with a history of chronic congestive heart failure and extreme obesity presents to the ED. She is alert but disoriented. Vital signs show pulse 143 beats/min, BP 145/94 mm Hg, oral temperature 37° C, and respirations 28 breaths/min shallow and labored. She has no cough. Breath sounds are decreased throughout with bilateral inspiratory coarse crackles. Electrocardiogram shows sinus tachycardia with a widened QRS complex and an occasional premature ventricular contraction. Her ABGs on a 50% air entrainment mask are pH 7.30, P_aCO_2 51 mm Hg, P_aO_2 50 mm Hg, S_aO_2 85%, and HCO_3^- 24 mEq/L. Which of the following should the respiratory therapist should recommend at this time?
   a. Nonrebreathing mask
   b. CPAP
   c. Intubation and mechanical ventilation
   d. Bilevel noninvasive positive pressure ventilation

6. An 18-year-old man is brought to the ED via ambulance following a serious bicycle crash with witnesses stating the patient was not wearing a helmet. The patient is unconscious and semiresponsive with a Glasgow Coma Score of 1/1/4 totaling 6. Vital signs show pulse 110 beats/min and regular, BP 96/55 mm Hg, oral temperature 36.6° C, and respirations 38 breaths/min and shallow with no cough. Chest auscultation reveals decreased breath sounds throughout. ABG results on a simple mask at 6 L/min are pH 7.22, P_aCO_2 58 mm Hg, P_aO_2 52 mm Hg, S_aO_2 76%, and HCO_3^- 22 mEq/L. Based on these findings the respiratory therapist should initiate which of the following?
   a. Nonrebreathing mask
   b. CPAP
   c. Intubation and mechanical ventilation
   d. Noninvasive positive pressure ventilation

7. A 135-pound patient with Guillain-Barré has been monitored in the ICU by the respiratory therapist over the past 6 hours. Both MIPs and vital capacity (VC) values have been recorded as follows:

Time	MIP	VC
7:00 AM	−40 cm H2O	3.1 L
9:15 AM	−35 cm H2O	2.8 L
11:25 AM	−25 cm H2O	1.5 L
1:10 PM	−15 cm H2O	0.64 L

Following the last assessment at 1:10 PM, what therapeutic intervention should the respiratory therapist recommend?
   a. 50% air entrainment mask
   b. CPAP
   c. Intubation and mechanical ventilation
   d. Noninvasive positive pressure ventilation

8. A 40-year-old woman presents to the ED with a 2-day history of dyspnea; productive cough with thick, green sputum; fever; and chills. The respiratory therapist's assessment reveals the following: pulse 105 beats/min, respirations 30 breaths/min, BP 132/84 mm Hg, oral temperature 39° C, decreased chest excursion of the right, and dull percussion over the right base. Chest auscultation indicates coarse crackles and wheezes over the right base. ABG results on room air reveal pH 7.35, P_aCO_2 31 mm Hg, P_aO_2 72 mm Hg, S_aO_2 88%, and HCO_3^- 24 mEq/L. The respiratory therapist should recommend which of the following?
   a. Nasal cannula at 4 L/min
   b. Continuous aerosol with 30% oxygen
   c. CPAP
   d. Noninvasive positive pressure ventilation

9. Which of the following conditions demonstrates the need for intubation and mechanical ventilation?
   a. Moderate hypoxemia
   b. ARF
   c. Chronic respiratory failure
   d. Hypoxic respiratory failure

10. A disorder that may cause hypercapnic respiratory failure because of increased work of breathing includes which of the following?
   a. Asthma
   b. Botulism
   c. Metabolic acidosis
   d. Cerebral hemorrhage

Chapter 4 Establishing the Need for Mechanical Ventilation

5 Selecting the Ventilator and the Mode

LEARNING OBJECTIVES

On completion of this chapter the reader will be able to do the following:

1. Select an appropriate mechanical ventilation mode based on findings derived from a patient's history and physical assessment.
2. Describe two methods of delivering noninvasive positive pressure ventilation.
3. Compare the advantages and disadvantages of volume-controlled and pressure-controlled ventilation.
4. Explain the differences in function between continuous mandatory ventilation (CMV), intermittent mandatory ventilation (IMV), and spontaneous ventilation.
5. Use the terms *trigger*, *cycle*, and *limit* to define volume-targeted CMV, pressure-targeted CMV, volume-targeted IMV, pressure-targeted IMV, and pressure-support ventilation (PSV).
6. Define each of the following terms: *pressure augmentation*, *pressure-regulated volume control* (PRVC), *volume support*, *mandatory minute ventilation* (MMV), *airway pressure release ventilation* (APRV), *bilevel positive airway pressure* (BiPAP), and *proportional assist ventilation* (PAV).
7. Give examples of the types of patients who would benefit most from each mode of ventilation.

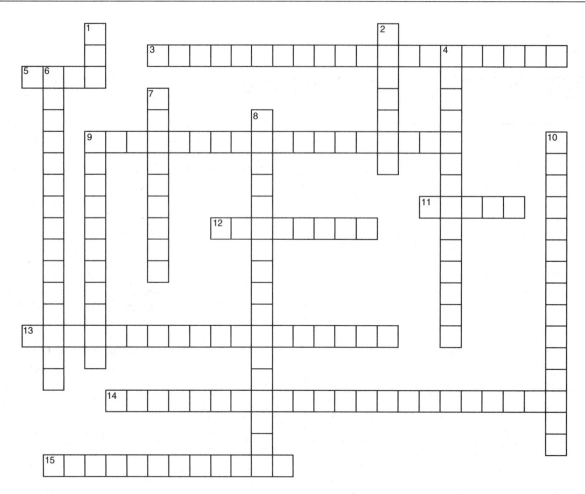

Across

3 Over ventilation in the CMV mode can cause this (two words)
5 A mode of ventilation that uses two levels of continuous positive airway pressure (CPAP) (abbreviation)
9 When the patient controls the timing and the tidal volume (two words)
11 Inverse ventilation with pressure control (abbreviation)
12 Type of control variable
13 Mode of ventilation with only time-triggered breaths (two words)
14 The ventilator supplies all the energy necessary to maintain alveolar ventilation (three words)
15 Occurs when the patient and the ventilator are not working together

Down

1 Mode of ventilation where all breaths are mandatory and can be volume or pressure targeted (abbreviation)
2 Type of ventilatory support where patient is participating in the work of breathing (WOB)
4 Patient-triggered volume or pressure-targeted ventilation (hyphenated word)
6 A mode that supports the spontaneously breathing patient to help reduce WOB (two words)
7 Type of breath where the timing and/or the tidal volume is controlled by the ventilator
8 Guarantees a specific volume delivery (two words)
9 The ventilator setting used to determine the ventilator response to the patient's inspiratory effort
10 A cross between mandatory and spontaneous breaths

Chapter **5** **Selecting the Ventilator and the Mode**

CHAPTER REVIEW QUESTIONS

1. List seven questions that the clinician should ask when determining the appropriate ventilator and mode of ventilation.

    a. _____

    b. _____

    c. _____

    d. _____

    e. _____

    f. _____

    g. _____

2. Match the appropriate ventilation support type with the appropriate ventilator connection or interface (there may be more than one answer):

    _____ Negative pressure ventilation   A. Oral endotracheal tube

    _____ CPAP   B. Nasal mask

    _____ Positive pressure ventilation   C. Face mask

       D. Chest cuirass

    _____ Noninvasive positive pressure ventilation   E. Tracheostomy tube

3. CPAP is commonly used in the hospital setting as a method to _____ while in the home-care setting it is typically used when treating

    _____

4. Acute-on-chronic respiratory failure is most often treated with which type of noninvasive positive pressure ventilation (NIV)? _____

5. Name a type of ventilation that reduces the requirements for heavy patient sedation.

    _____

6. List five disorders that are sometimes managed with NIV.

    a. _____

    b. _____

    c. _____

    d. _____

    e. _____

7. List both advantages and disadvantages of NIV in a patient with acute respiratory failure.

Advantage	Disadvantage
_____	_____
_____	_____
_____	_____
_____	_____
_____	_____

8. Define the terms *full ventilatory support* (FVS) and *partial ventilatory support* (PVS).

    _____

    _____

    _____

9. The typical minimum ventilatory rate setting for a patient receiving FVS is considered _____ breaths/min.

10. PVS typically uses set machine rates of lower than

    _____ breaths/min with the patient participating in the WOB to help maintain effective alveolar ventilation.

11. What type of ventilatory support would you consider using when your patient has acute ventilatory failure from ventilatory muscle fatigue or a high WOB? Why?

    _____

    _____

    _____

12. List and explain the three types of breath delivery.

    a. _____

    b. _____

    c. _____

13. What is the primary advantage of volume-control ventilation?

    _____

14. What is the main disadvantage of volume-control ventilation?

    _____

15. During volume-control ventilation a patient develops acute bronchospasm. What will happen to (a) the peak inspiratory pressure? Why? What will happen to (b) the amount of volume delivered to the patient? Why?

    a. _____

    _____

    b. _____

    _____

16. A patient experiencing acute bronchospasm receives an adrenergic bronchodilator. If the bronchodilator is effective, the peak inspiratory pressure is expected

    to _____. Why? _____

    _____

17. When targeting pressure as the control variable, what will vary with changing lung characteristics?

    _____

18. What are three advantages of pressure-control ventilation (PCV)?

    a. _____

    b. _____

    c. _____

19. What are three disadvantages of PCV?

    a. _____

    b. _____

    c. _____

20. When a patient's lung compliance worsens during PCV, what will happen to tidal volume being

    delivered? _____

21. What are the three types of breath delivery timing or sequence available on current Intensive Care Unit (ICU) ventilators? Briefly describe each.

    a. _____

    b. _____

    c. _____

22. What three characteristics determine the mode of ventilation?

    a. _____

    b. _____

    c. _____

23. List the five basic modes of ventilation.

    a. _____

    b. _____

    c. _____

    d. _____

    e. _____

24. How should clinicians differentiate between controlled and assisted ventilation?

    _____

25. Give a clinical situation where assist-controlled ventilation is appropriate?

    _____

    _____

    _____

26. What happens when the clinician inappropriately sets ventilator sensitivity?

    _____

    _____

27. What two triggers can begin inspiration in patient-triggered assisted ventilation?

    a. _____

    b. _____

28. Studies have shown that vital capacity (VC)-CMV may actually increase the patient's WOB by

    _____ %. How is this observed in the clinical setting? How is this corrected?

    _____

29. What settings are typically set by the clinician in PC-CMV?

    _____

    _____

30. What determines the tidal volume delivered in PC-CMV?

_____

31. What flow-curve type has been shown to improve gas distribution and allow the patient to vary inspiratory gas flow during spontaneous breathing efforts?

_____

32. A safety mechanism to avoid excessive system pressure is the _____ and is set at about _____ above the set pressure level and will cause _____ to end when reached.

33. Describe a clinical scenario where pressure control inverse ratio ventilation (PC-IRV) would be appropriate?

_____

_____

34. Explain how IMV differs from CMV?

_____

_____

_____

35. Fill in the table below regarding the advantages, risks, and disadvantages of CMV and IMV.

Mode	Advantages	Risks and Disadvantages
VC-CMV or PC-CMV	_____	_____
	_____	_____
	_____	_____
	_____	_____
	_____	_____
	_____	_____
	_____	_____
	_____	_____
	_____	_____
VC-IMV or PC-IMV	_____	_____
	_____	_____
	_____	_____
	_____	_____
	_____	_____
	_____	_____
	_____	_____
	_____	_____

36. What is the goal when choosing IMV mode for a patient?

_____

_____

37. What are the three basic means of providing support for continuous spontaneous breathing during mechanical ventilation?

   a. _____

   b. _____

   c. _____

38. Briefly describe a spontaneous breathing trial.

_____

_____

39. What patient characteristics are necessary for PSV to be successful?

_____

_____

_____

40. What ventilator parameters are set by the clinician in PSV? What parameters does the patient establish?

_____

41. What determines tidal volume in PSV?

_____

_____

42. What situation can cause the ventilator in the PSV mode to time cycle?

_____

43. Define the term *rise time*.

_____

44. Inspiration is _____ cycled in PSV.

45. Give a clinical scenario where patients may require a shorter inspiratory time.

_____

46. What pressure levels does a clinician set in bilevel pressure assist?

_____

47. What patient variables can end inspiration in the bilevel pressure-assist mode?

_____

48. What patient characteristic can influence the specific time and pressure limits used during PSV?

_____

49. Explain how pressure augmentation (P_{Aug}) works? What is an alternate term used to describe $P_{(aug)}$?

_____

_____

_____

50. In P_{Aug}, if the set volume is achieved prior to flow cycling, what will happen to the breath?

_____

51. In P_{Aug}, if the set volume is not reached before flow drops to the set level, how will the ventilator respond?

_____

_____

52. Describe a clinical scenario where a patient can receive more volume than is set by the clinician in P_{Aug}?

_____

_____

_____

53. Describe PRVC in terms of trigger, limit, and cycle.

_____

54. Fill in the table below regarding the different proprietary names given to PRVC.

Ventilator	PRVC name
CareFusion Avea	•
Covidien PB 840	•
Hamilton G5 and G3	•
Dräger Evita XL	•
Servo-i	•

55. Generally, at what pressure will a ventilator alarm while in the PRVC mode if the upper pressure limit is set at 40 cm H_2O and the tidal volume is set at 600 mL?

_____

_____

56. Describe volume-support ventilation (VSV) in terms of trigger, limit, and cycle.

_____

_____

57. What is the difference between PRVC and VSV?

_____

_____

_____

58. Define MMV. _____

_____

59. In MVV, what alarms must be set to protect against problems associated with rapid, shallow breathing?

_____

_____

60. The mode of ventilation that requires two levels of CPAP and allows the patient to breath spontaneously at both levels is known as

_____.

61. The optimum duration of the release time for the mode mentioned in Question 60 is a function of the

_____ of the respiratory system.

62. APRV was originally intended to ventilate patients

with _____.

63. With PAV, what three variables are proportional to the patient's spontaneous effort?

_____

_____

64. In PAV mode what two factors determine the amount of pressure produced by the ventilator?

a. _____

b. _____

65. What are the advantages and disadvantages of PAV?

_____

_____

_____

_____

CRITICAL THINKING QUESTIONS

1. A patient is waking up following surgery and is currently receiving mechanical ventilation in the PC-CMV mode. During rounds the respiratory therapist observes the patient's use of accessory muscles, diaphoresis, patient-ventilator asynchrony, and no assisted breaths. What is the most probable source of this patient's clinical appearance? How can this be corrected?

_____

_____

_____

_____

_____

2. If a patient's ventilatory drive increases during the use of VC-CMV, what changes will occur to the patient's acid-base balance? What can be done to regulate this?

_____

_____

_____

_____

3. Which mode of ventilation would a home-care patient with central sleep apnea benefit from and why?

_____

_____

_____

_____

_____

4. Match the patient condition with a ventilator mode most likely to benefit the patient.

Patient with the following:

_____ (1) Intubated with quadriplegia from a spinal cord injury
_____ (2) Intubated with acute respiratory distress syndrome
_____ (3) Obstructive sleep apnea in the home-care setting
_____ (4) Intubated with spontaneous breathing with acute lung injury
_____ (5) Intubated with consistent spontaneous respiratory pattern
_____ (6) Nonintubated spontaneously breathing with refractory hypoxemia
_____ (7) Intubated with drug overdose

Would benefit from this ventilator mode:

a. Nasal mask CPAP
b. CPAP through ventilator
c. Pressure support
d. VC-CMV
e. PC-CMV with positive end-expiratory pressure (PEEP)

CASE STUDIES

Case Study 1

In the ICU the respiratory therapist approaches a patient receiving mechanical ventilation. The ventilator monitor shows the following scalar.

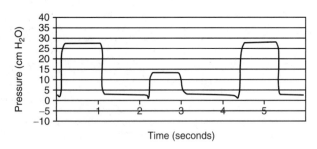

Time (seconds)

1. What mode of ventilation is the ventilator set to deliver?

_____

2. What is the inspiratory time for the mechanical breaths?

_____

3. What is the ventilator expiratory time?

_____

Case Study 2

A 6-foot 3-inch male patient who was involved in a motor vehicle crash (MVC) arrives in the emergency department with chest and facial injuries. Because of the nature of the facial injuries, he is intubated with a size 8.0 mm endotracheal tube. Following resuscitative measures he is transferred to the ICU.

1. What type of ventilator support would this patient require initially?

_____

2. What ventilator mode would you use when this patient wakes, has the desire to breathe spontaneously, and has a P_aO_2 of 58 mm Hg with the F_IO_2 set at 0.50?

_____

Case Study 3

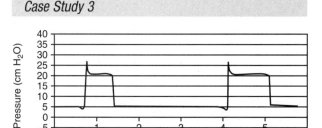

Time (seconds)

1. What mode of ventilation does Figure 5-2 represent?

_____

2. Identify the issue with this pressure tracing.

_____

3. What can be done to resolve the identified problem?

_____

NBRC-STYLE QUESTIONS

1. When switching from the CMV mode to the IMV mode to facilitate weaning from mechanical ventilation, which of the following could be used, in addition to IMV (IMV), to assist in this process?
   a. PCV
   b. PSV
   c. PAV
   d. APRV

2. A post-thoracic surgery patient currently receiving mechanical ventilation on VC-CMV with 60% oxygen has the following arterial blood gas (ABG): pH 7.45, P_aCO_2 36 mm Hg, P_aO_2 68 mm Hg. The patient's peak inspiratory pressures are averaging 55 cm H_2O. The ventilator mode that is most appropriate at this time is which of the following?
   a. PSV
   b. VC-IMV with PEEP
   c. PC-CMV with PEEP
   d. MMV

3. A 38-year-old female suffered a deceleration injury in an MVC. She is alert and oriented but in respiratory distress. A portion of the patient's right anterior chest wall is moving in a paradoxical motion. Breath sounds are decreased on the right and the trachea is midline and no pneumothorax was detected. ABG data reveal pH 7.48, P_aCO_2 31 mm Hg, P_aO_2 63 mm Hg, and HCO_3^- 24 mEq/L. The respiratory therapist should recommend which of the following therapies for this patient at this time?
   a. Mask CPAP with supplemental oxygen
   b. Intubate and use VC-CMV with PEEP
   c. NIV with supplemental oxygen
   d. Intubate and use PCIRV

4. The physician requests that the respiratory therapist make a recommendation for a patient with postpolio complaints of increasing daytime weakness. Her VC is 12 mL/kg and maximal inspiratory pressure is −32 cm H_2O. Her ABG on room air reveals pH 7.38, P_aCO_2 46 mm Hg, P_aO_2 74 mm Hg, and HCO_3^- 24 mEq/L. The respiratory therapist should suggest which of the following?
   a. Tracheostomy with PSV
   b. Tracheostomy with VC-CMV
   c. BiPAP via nasal mask at night
   d. Full face mask CPAP with supplemental oxygen

5. During a pressure-triggered breath in VC-CMV the pressure-time curve on the graphic display does not rise smoothly and appears to be somewhat concave in appearance. This indicates which of the following?
   a. Flow rate is inadequate
   b. Rise time is set too slow
   c. Overshoot on the pressure
   d. Inspiratory time is too short

6. Every breath from the ventilator is time or patient triggered, pressure targeted (limited), and time cycled. This describes which of the following ventilator modes?
   a. PAug
   b. APRV
   c. PCV
   d. VC-IMV

7. Pressure augmentation (PAug) may be beneficial for mechanically ventilated patients with which of the following?
   1. Noncardiogenic pulmonary edema
   2. Acute Respiratory Distress Syndrome
   3. Postoperative upper abdominal surgery
   4. Receiving heavy sedation and paralyzing agents
   a. 1 and 2 only
   b. 1 and 3 only
   c. 2 and 4 only
   d. 3 and 4 only

8. The ventilator mode that allows the patient to breathe spontaneously at two levels of positive pressure is known as which of the following?
   a. CPAP
   b. PAug
   c. PRVC
   d. APRV

9. A patient is intubated and on PSV. The respiratory therapist notices that inspiratory time has increased from 1 second to 2 seconds consistently on every breath since last ventilator rounds. What should be the first action the respiratory therapist should do to correct the problem?
   a. Change to the SIMV mode
   b. Check the endotracheal tube cuff pressure
   c. Increase the inspiratory flow setting
   d. Suction and lavage the patient's airway

10. When lung compliance decreases while a patient is receiving mechanical ventilation with PCV which of the will occur?
    a. Peak pressure will increase.
    b. Peak pressure will decrease.
    c. Tidal volume will increase.
    d. Tidal volume will decrease.

HELPFUL INTERNET SITES

- A. Jones, "Current Ventilation Modes & Controls" http://www.respiratorycare-online.com/lecture_series/vent_modes/current_vent_modes_handout.pdf
- P.J. David, "A Primer on Mechanical Ventilation," MED 610: Clinical Respiratory Diseases & Critical Care Medicine, Seattle http://courses.washington.edu/med610/mechanical-ventilation/mv_primer.html
- Hamilton Medical, Hamilton G5 Online Simulation http://www.hamilton-medical.com/Online-simulation.683.0.html

6 Initial Ventilator Settings

LEARNING OBJECTIVES

On completion of this chapter the reader will be able to do the following:

1. Calculate minute ventilation given a patient's respiratory rate and tidal volume.
2. Calculate total cycle time, inspiratory time, expiratory time, flow in L/s, and inspiratory-to-expiratory ratios (I:E) given the necessary patient data.
3. Select an appropriate flow rate and pattern.
4. Calculate initial minute ventilation, tidal volume, and rate for a patient placed on vital capacity (VC)-continuous mandatory ventilation (CMV) based on the patient's sex, height, and ideal body weight (IBW).
5. Identify the source of the problem when an inspiratory pause cannot be measured.
6. Choose an appropriate initial mode of mechanical ventilation, determine V_E, tidal volume, frequency (rate), and positive end-expiratory pressure (PEEP) settings based on the patient's lung pathology, body temperature, metabolic rate, altitude, and acid-base balance.
7. Evaluate the response in peak inspiratory pressure (PIP) and plateau pressure when the flow waveform is changed.
8. Recommend the selection and initial settings for the various modes of pressure-controlled ventilation (PCV), including bilevel positive airway pressure (BiPAP), pressure support ventilation (PSV), PCV, and Servo-controlled (dual modes) ventilation.
9. Identify a problem in PSV from a pressure-time graph.
10. Measure plateau pressure using pressure-time and flow-time waveforms during pressure-controlled mechanical ventilation.
11. List the possible causes for a change in pressure during pressure-regulated volume control (PRVC).
12. Identify the mode of ventilation based on the trigger, target, and cycle criteria.

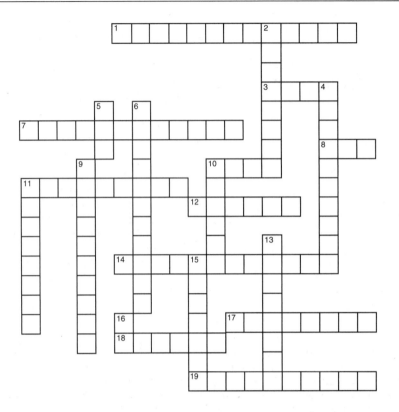

Across

1 Too much pressure in the alveoli can cause this
3 The abbreviation for a pressure-limited, time-cycled mode that uses the set tidal volume as a feedback control
7 Airway resistance multiplied by lung compliance is one _____ (two words)
8 The type of ventilation used to augment spontaneous breathing in patients with artificial airways (abbreviation)
10 The name of the type of flow waveform that represents the tapered flow at the end of inspiratory phase
11 A type of flow pattern created by a progressive increase in flow during inspiration
12 The chart used to determine body surface area (BSA)
14 The type of volume that is lost in the patient circuit
17 The Dräger V500 calls its volume support by this name
18 The brand of ventilator that has no flow waveform selector or peak flow control
19 The type of flow waveform that occurs naturally in pressure ventilation

Down

2 On the Hamilton G5 ventilator, PRVC is called _____ pressure ventilation
4 To calculate how much volume is lost in the patient circuit tubing, _____ must be known
5 One entire breathing cycle (abbreviation)
6 The type of pause used to measure plateau pressure
9 Adding tubing to the patient's endotracheal tube will add this type of dead space
10 A constant flow pattern produces this type of flow waveform
11 Air trapping is measured as this
13 The amount of inspiratory time required for the ventilator to reach the set pressure at the beginning of inspiration (two words)
15 The nomogram used to obtain ventilator settings
16 A purely spontaneous mode in which the operator sets the ventilator sensitivity, tidal volume, and upper pressure limit (abbreviation)

Chapter **6** **Initial Ventilator Settings**

CHAPTER REVIEW QUESTIONS

1. The primary goal of mechanical ventilation is to achieve a _____ that matches the patient's needs.

2. In a healthy person what is the typical oxygen consumption and the carbon dioxide consumption? What is the abbreviation used for each?

3. Metabolic rate is directly related to _____ and _____ in humans.

4. List eight parameters to consider when setting a patient up for assist-control volume-controlled ventilation.

   a. _____   e. _____

   b. _____   f. _____

   c. _____   g. _____

   d. _____   h. _____

Questions 5 through 7 refer to Figure 6-1.

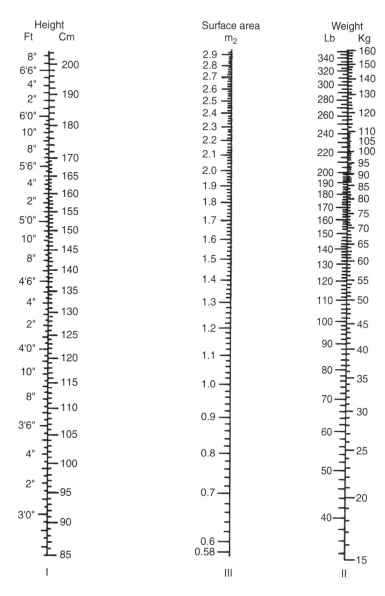

5. Find the BSA for a person who weighs 200 pounds and is 6 feet 2 inches tall.

_____

6. Find the BSA for a person who weighs 75 kg and is 155 cm tall.

_____

7. Find the BSA for a person who weighs 178 pounds and is 5 feet 7 inches tall.

_____

Questions 8 through 11: Calculate minute ventilation for the following individuals.

Question	Gender	BSA	Body Temp.	Comment	Minute Ventilation
8.	F	1.6 m^2	39°C	N/A	_____
9.	M	2.8 m^2	37°C	6000 ft above sea level	_____
10.	M	2.3 m^2	101°F	N/A	_____
11.	F	1.9 m^2	98.6°F	Metabolic acidosis	_____

12. The initial tidal volume setting for adults should be within what range? _____

13. The initial tidal volume setting for infants and children should be within what range? _____

14. The estimated V_T range for a female patient that has an IBW of 50 kg is _____.

15. The estimated V_T range for a male patient with an IBW of 90 kg is _____.

16. What is the normal V_T range for a spontaneously breathing patient?

_____

17. What is the normal range for the respiratory rate in a spontaneously breathing patient?

_____

18. Recommend the initial tidal volume, respiratory rate, and minute ventilation for a 5-foot 2-inch tall female who has just arrived in the postoperative care unit.

_____

_____

_____

19. Recommend the initial tidal volume, respiratory rate, and minute ventilation for a 71-inch tall male with chronic obstructive pulmonary disease (COPD).

_____

_____

_____

20. Recommend the initial tidal volume, respiratory rate, and minute ventilation for a 69-inch male with pulmonary fibrosis.

_____

_____

_____

21. Calculate and fill in the missing information.

Tidal Volume	Respiratory Rate	Minute Ventilation
a. 750 mL	12 breaths/min	_____
b. 580 mL	10 breaths/min	_____
c. _____	15 breaths/min	6.9 L/min
d. _____	20 breaths/min	8.3 L/min
e. 460 mL	_____	5.2 L/min
f. 660 mL	_____	9.5 L/min

22. Calculate the total cycle time (TCT) for the following frequencies (e.g., rate setting).

    a. 30 breaths/min _____

    b. 15 breaths/min _____

    c. 12 breaths/min _____

    d. 10 breaths/min _____

23. Use the corresponding frequencies in Question 22 to calculate the expiratory time (T_E) for each of the given inspiratory times (T_I).

    a. T_I = 1 second _____

    b. T_I = 0.75 second _____

    c. T_I = 1.25 seconds _____

    d. T_I = 2 seconds _____

24. Use the corresponding information from Question 23 to determine I:E ratios.

    a. _____

    b. _____

    c. _____

    d. _____

25. Calculate the T_I, T_E, and TCT given and I:E ratio of 1:3 and rate = 12 beats/min.

26. Calculate the T_I, T_E, and TCT given an I:E ratio of 1:2 and rate = 25 beats/min.

27. Calculate V_T given T_I = 1 second and a flow of 50 L/min.

28. Calculate T_I given $V_T = 700$ mL and a flow of 50 L/min.

_____

_____

29. Increasing the set flow rate while ventilating an apneic patient in VC-CMV will cause the T_I to

_____, the PIP to _____, and

the gas distribution to _____.

30. What are the guidelines for setting T_I, I:E ratio, and flow rates during CMV?

_____

31. The type of flow waveform pattern created by pressure ventilation is

_____

32. The flow waveform that creates the highest PIP during volume ventilation, when R_{aw} is elevated, is

_____

33. The flow waveform(s) most appropriate for normal

lungs is (are) _____

34. Why is a descending flow pattern beneficial for patients with hypoxemia and low lung compliance?

_____

_____

_____

_____

35. What is an inspiratory pause most frequently used to determine?

_____

36. The respiratory therapist attempts to measure plateau pressure by adding a 1-second inspiratory pause. The set VC-CMV rate is 12, the current rate is 20, and the plateau pressure is unattainable. What is the most likely cause of this problem?

_____

_____

37. The pressure ventilation modes that have time triggering include

_____

38. The pressure ventilation modes that allow for patient triggering include

_____.

39. Flow cycling is used by which pressure ventilation modes?

_____

40. Time cycling is used by which pressure ventilation modes?

_____

41. What are the advantages and disadvantages of using pressure ventilation?

_____

_____

_____

_____

42. Explain the concept of using low PEEP levels for patients with COPD.

_____

_____

_____

_____

43. During pressure ventilation, how is tidal volume established?

_____

44. A patient on PC-CMV has a PIP setting of 18 cm H_2O. The V_T is measured as 400 mL. The desired V_T is 750 mL. How should the pressure be adjusted to achieve the desired V_T?

_____

_____

_____

45. A patient on PC-CMV has a set PIP of 14 cm H_2O. The exhaled V_T measured is 550 mL. The desired exhaled V_T is 800 mL. How should the pressure be adjusted to achieve the desired volume?

_____

_____

46. What formula can be used to estimate the level of pressure support needed for a patient?

_____

_____

47. During VC-CMV the settings are as follows: f = 12 breaths/min, V_T = 600 mL. The patient's PIP was measured at 28 cm H_2O with a $P_{plateau}$ of 20 cm H_2O. The patient is now ready for VC-intermittent mandatory ventilation (IMV) with pressure support. Recommend an appropriate level to start this patient's pressure support at during this mode of ventilation.

_____

48. Refer to Figure 6-2. Identify the problem on the pressure-time graph of a COPD patient receiving CPAP +5 cm H_2O with pressure support ventilation.

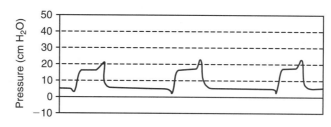

_____

49. What can be done to correct the identified problem in Question 48?

_____

50. The flow cycling percentage is set to 20% and the peak inspiratory flow is 50 L/min. At what flow rate will the ventilator cycle to exhalation?

_____

51. The flow cycling percentage is set to 40% and the peak inspiratory flow is 50 L/min. At what flow rate will the ventilator cycle to exhalation?

_____

52. Compare the answers for Questions 50 and 51. Which flow cycling set percentage will provide the shortest inspiratory time? Explain your answer.

_____

_____

53. What are the three ways of establishing the initial PIP during PCV?

    a. _____

    b. _____

    c. _____

54. a. What are the initial setting ranges for BiPAP?

    b. What is the target tidal volume during BiPAP?

    a. _____

    b. _____

55. The ventilator mode where the breath is pressure limited, time cycled, and uses V_T as a feedback control is

_____

56. How does the Servo-i establish initial pressure in the PRVC mode?

_____

_____

57. Why is it important to set an upper pressure limit during PRVC?

_____

_____

_____

58. During ventilation of a patient with PRVC the respiratory therapist notes there is an audible alarm and a digital message that says "pressure limit, please evaluate." List four causes of this problem.

_____

_____

59. Explain how P_{alv} is estimated during PC-CMV.

_____

_____

CRITICAL THINKING QUESTIONS

1. What considerations need to be made by the respiratory therapist before initiating mechanical ventilation?

_____

_____

_____

2. How do changes in compliance affect the airway pressure and exhaled tidal volume in the volume-control mode compared to the pressure-control mode?

_____

_____

_____

3. What two safety systems do ventilators have to end inspiration during PSV?

_____

_____

_____

CASE STUDIES

Case Study

A 28-year-old woman presents to the emergency department with complaints of difficulty breathing, general muscle weakness, and dysphagia. Her history of present illness reveals that she was diagnosed with infectious mononucleosis 10 days ago and has recently experienced ptosis and weakness in her legs and arms. She weighs 150 pounds and is 5 feet 8 inches tall. Arterial blood gas analysis on room air reveals pH 7.30, P_aCO_2 50 mm Hg, PO_2 78 mm Hg, S_aO_2 91%, and HCO_3^- 23 mEq/L. Her maximal inspiratory pressure is 15 cm H_2O and VC is 13 mL/kg.

1. What is the most appropriate action at this time?

_____

2. Calculate the patient's minute ventilation using the Dubois Body Surface Chart in Figure 6-1.

_____

3. What tidal volume and respiratory rate ranges would be appropriate for this patient?

_____

Fifteen minutes later the patient's breathing is very shallow; she is unresponsive and is immediately intubated.

4. Suggest an appropriate mode of ventilation for this patient? Explain your choice.

_____

5. What ventilator settings would you recommend?

_____

NBRC-STYLE QUESTIONS

1. A 6-foot tall male patient with pulmonary fibrosis is being ventilated in VC-CMV, rate 10 breaths/min, VT 600 mL, F_IO_2 0.50, and PEEP +10 cm H_2O. The patient's PIP is 53 cm H_2O, and the $P_{plateau}$ is 47 cm H_2O. It is decided to switch the patient to PC-CMV. What set PIP will deliver 6 mL/kg IBW?
   a. 30 cm H_2O
   b. 35 cm H_2O
   c. 38 cm H_2O
   d. 43 cm H_2O

2. The most appropriate initial settings for a 5-foot 4-inch tall female postoperative patient with no lung disease would be which of the following?
   a. PC-CMV, PIP 35 cm H_2O, f 20 breaths/min, PEEP +10 cm H_2O
   b. PC-SIMV, PIP 20 cm H_2O, f 6 breaths/min, PEEP +8 cm H_2O
   c. VC-CMV, 450 mL, f 10 breaths/min, PEEP +5 cm H_2O
   d. VC-CMV, 700 mL, f 14 breaths/min, PEEP 0 cm H_2O

3. A patient is ready to be changed from VC-IMV to PSV. The VC-IMV settings were VT 450 mL, f 4 breaths/min, and PEEP +5 cm H_2O. The patient's PIP is 31 cm H_2O, and $P_{plateau}$ is 23 cm H_2O. The initial PSV setting for this patient should be which of the following?
   a. 5 cm H_2O
   b. 8 cm H_2O
   c. 10 cm H_2O
   d. 12 cm H_2O

4. The flow waveform that is most appropriate for a patient with high R_{aw} is which of the following?
   a. Rectangle
   b. Descending
   c. Ascending
   d. Exponential

5. Calculate the I:E ratio when the set rate is 35 breaths/min and the T_I = 1 second.
   a. 1:1
   b. 1.4:1
   c. 1.7:1
   d. 2:1

6. What flow rate is necessary to deliver a V_T 500 mL at a rate of 15 breaths/min with an I:E ratio of 1:3?
   a. 30 L/min
   b. 35 L/min
   c. 40 L/min
   d. 45 L/min

7. The appropriate minute ventilation for a male with a BSA of 2.3 m^2 and a body temperature of 40°C is which of the following?
   a. 8.2 L/min
   b. 9.6 L/min
   c. 10.6 L/min
   d. 11.7 L/min

8. A 5-foot 1-inch tall female patient receiving PSV 6 cm H_2O is showing signs of accessory muscle use and is exhaling a V_T of 220 mL at a rate of 28 breaths/min. The most appropriate action at this time is which of the following?
   a. Adjust the FIO_2.
   b. Increase the set flow rate.
   c. Increase the PSV to 10 cm H_2O.
   d. Adjust the flow cycling percent.

9. A 5-foot 7-inch tall female multiple trauma patient was being managed on VC-CMV, f 12 breaths/min, V_T 640 mL, PEEP +5 cm H_2O, F_IO_2 60%, and a constant waveform for the past 24 hours. Currently, PIP is 45 cm H_2O, $P_{plateau}$ is 38 cm H_2O, and the patient has been diagnosed with acute respiratory distress syndrome. The respiratory therapist wants to switch the patient to PC-CMV. The initial pressure setting to target the appropriate V_T for this patient is which of the following?
   a. 10 cm H_2O
   b. 20 cm H_2O
   c. 38 cm H_2O
   d. 45 cm H_2O

10. How is pressure support ventilation cycled?
    a. Flow
    b. Pressure
    c. Volume
    d. Time

HELPFUL INTERNET SITES

- G.R.S. Budinger, "Mechanical Ventilation." A Power-Point presentation available on LUMEN summarizing many aspects of mechanical ventilation.
http://www.lumen.luc.edu/lumen/MedEd/medicine/pulmonar/lecture/vent/case_f.htm
- "AARC–Adult Mechanical Ventilator Protocols." American Association for Respiratory Care.
http://www.aarc.org/resources/protocol_resources/documents/general_vent.pdf

- D.J. Pierson, "A Primer on Mechanical Ventilation," MED 610 Clinical Respiratory Diseases & Critical Care Medicine, Seattle
http://courses.washington.edu/med610/mechanical-ventilation/mv_primer.html

Final Considerations in Ventilator Setup

LEARNING OBJECTIVES

Upon completion of this chapter, the reader will be able to do the following:

1. Recommend fractional inspired oxygen concentration (F_IO_2) settings when initiating mechanical ventilation.
2. Discuss the pros and cons of using the sigh function during mechanical ventilation.
3. Compare the use of sigh with the concept of a recruitment maneuver in Acute Respiratory Distress Syndrome (ARDS).
4. List the actions necessary for final ventilator setup.
5. Explain the concept of using extrinsic positive end-expiratory pressure (PEEP) in patients with airflow obstruction and air trapping who have trouble triggering a breath during mechanical ventilation.
6. Calculate the desired F_IO_2 setting given the current partial arterial pressure of oxygen (PaO_2) and F_IO_2 values.
7. List the essential capabilities of an adult intensive care unit (ICU) ventilator.
8. Provide initial ventilator settings from the guidelines for patient management for any of the following patient conditions: chronic obstructive pulmonary disease (COPD), acute asthma episodes, neuromuscular disorders, closed head injuries, ARDS, and acute cardiogenic pulmonary edema.

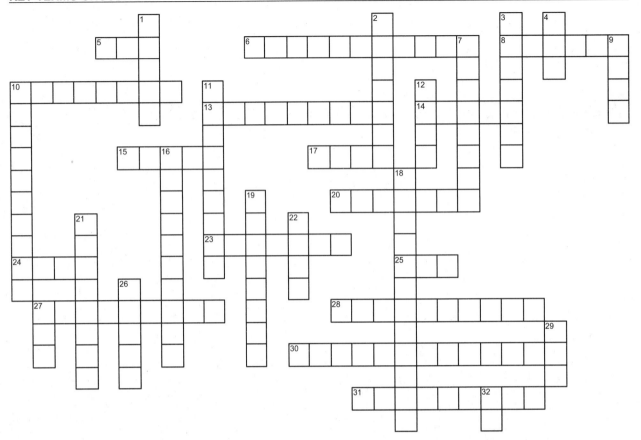

Across

5 A type of pressure measured to determine brain swelling in a patient with a closed head injury (abbreviation)
6 Pharmacologic agent that can improve myocardial oxygenation and reduce preload and afterload
8 The typical color of sputum in the presence of respiratory infection
10 The sound sometimes associated with alveoli popping open during inspiration
13 A pharmacologic agent given to improve cardiac contractility
14 Warn of possible dangers
15 Too much air in the lungs causes this type of resonance
17 The preferred method of patient trigger that has a rapid response time
20 Type of water with which a humidifier is filled
23 The normal response to acute increases in intracranial pressure (ICP)
24 A chemical administered to keep pH in an acceptable range (abbreviation)
25 The pressure required to maintain cerebral blood flow (abbreviation)
27 The process of adding fluids
28 Excess pressure in the lungs can cause this
30 Not in sync
31 Low amount of oxygen in the blood

Down

1 Type of alarm that warns when the patient stops breathing
2 Type of score used to evaluate a patient's neurologic responses
3 Type of hyperinflation that occurs with auto-PEEP
4 The neuromuscular disease that was made famous by a ball player (abbreviation)
7 A percentage of absolute humidity compared to capacity
9 A humidifier that uses capillary action
10 Presence of this in the circuit tubing can potentially be a source of accidental lavage
11 Type of medications given to reduce vascular fluid load
12 Interface for noninvasive ventilation
16 Knowingly allowing carbon dioxide levels to rise during mechanical ventilation is known as _____ hypercapnia
18 A look-and-see type of pulmonary diagnostic procedure
19 One type of humidifier
21 Type of deficit that increases when dry gas is inhaled
22 This type of breath is used for lung recruitment
26 Type of alarm that warns when inspiratory time exceeds expiratory time
27 An artificial nose (abbreviation)
29 The point at which inhaled air reaches 100% relative humidity (abbreviation)
32 A neuromuscular disease with rapid onset (abbreviation)

CHAPTER REVIEW QUESTIONS

1. The clinically acceptable arterial oxygen tension range is _____ .

2. Before elective intubation, a patient's partial pressure of arterial oxygen (P_aO_2) was 92 mm Hg with a nasal cannula running at 2 L/min. What F_IO_2 should be set on the ventilator? _____

3. Calculate the estimated F_IO_2 using the following information: known F_IO_2 0.50, known P_aO_2 60 mm Hg, desired P_aO_2 90 mm Hg.

   _____

   _____

   _____

4. What is the acceptable goal for pulse oximetry saturation (S_pO_2)?

   _____

5. Typically, how long following initiation of mechanical ventilation should a blood gas be drawn on a patient?

   _____

6. List three problems associated with the use of high concentrations of oxygen.

   a. _____

   b. _____

   c. _____

7. Why does flow triggering have a faster response time than pressure triggering?

   _____

   _____

   _____

8. Explain how auto-PEEP interferes with pressure triggering?

   _____

   _____

   _____

   _____

9. The point in the tracheobronchial tree at which inhaled gas contains 44 mg/L of water, has reached 100% relative humidity, and is 37°C is called the

   _____ and is located at the level of the

   _____ .

10. The absolute humidity of a ventilator's humidification system needs to be _____ at temperatures between _____ and _____ .

11. List two advantages of a closed humidification system.

    a. _____

    b. _____

12. Explain what causes excessive rain-out (condensation) in a ventilator circuit.

    _____

    _____

    _____

    _____

13. How much water can a heat moisture exchanger (HME) provide during tidal volumes of 500 to 1000 mL?

    _____

14. How much water can a hygroscopic HME provide during tidal volumes of 500 to 1000 mL?

    _____

15. What happens to an HME when moisture and secretions accumulate in it?

    _____

    _____

16. What should be done with the HME during an aerosol treatment using a small volume nebulizer? How can this be avoided?

    _____

    _____

    _____

17. A metered-dose inhaler with a spacer should be placed where in a ventilator circuit? What should be done with the HME?

_____

_____

_____

18. List five contraindications for the use of HMEs.

a. _____

b. _____

c. _____

d. _____

e. _____

19. List and explain the three levels of alarms that can happen during mechanical ventilation.

a. _____

b. _____

c. _____

For Questions 20 through 35, identify the alarm situations with the appropriate alarm level. **Select 1, 2, or 3**.

20. _____ Heater/humidifier malfunction

21. _____ Timing failure

22. _____ Autocycling

23. _____ Intrinsic PEEP

24. _____ Excessive gas delivery to patient

25. _____ Inappropriate PEEP/continuous positive airway pressure (CPAP)

26. _____ Exhalation valve failure

27. _____ Inspiratory-to-expiratory ratio (I:E ratio) inappropriate

28. _____ Electrical power failure

29. _____ Changes in lung characteristics

30. _____ Circuit leak

31. _____ No gas delivery to patient

32. _____ Electrical power failure

33. _____ Circuit partially obstructed

34. _____ Inappropriate oxygen level

35. _____ Changes in ventilatory drive

36. Following the application of vital capacity (VC)-continuous mandatory ventilation (CMV) with +8 cm H_2O PEEP to a patient, the respiratory therapist notices that the average peak inspiratory pressure (PIP) is 30 cm H_2O. What values would you suggest for the low-pressure, high-pressure, and low PEEP/CPAP alarms to be set?

_____

37. The maximum value at which the apnea alarm should be set with any ventilator is how many seconds?

_____

38. Describe the similarity between lung recruitment strategies and sigh maneuvers.

_____

_____

_____

39. List four circumstances where sighs or deep breaths are appropriate.

a. _____

b. _____

c. _____

d. _____

40. List the 10 steps the respiratory therapist should perform on the ventilator and other related equipment during the final preparation of ventilator set up.

a. _____

b. _____

c. _____

d. _____

e. _____

f. _____

g. _____

h. _____

i. _____

j. _____

41. Once the decision has been made to place a patient on mechanical ventilation, what steps should the respiratory therapist take?

a. _____

b. _____

c. _____

d. _____

e. _____

f. _____

42. List the essential capabilities of an adult ventilator.

a. Modes: _____

b. Tidal volume range: _____

c. Respiratory rate range: _____

d. Pressure range: _____

e. PEEP/CPAP range: _____

f. Flow rate range: _____

g. Flow waveforms: _____

h. F_IO_2: _____

i. Diagnostic measurements: _____

j. Alarms: _____

43. What lung characteristics do patients with COPD typically exhibit?

_____

44. What is the primary reason for mechanical ventilatory support for patients with COPD?

_____

45. List five causes of increased morbidity for COPD patients receiving mechanical ventilation.

a. _____

b. _____

c. _____

d. _____

e. _____

46. The guidelines for mechanical ventilation of COPD patients suggest which mode of choice, if possible?

_____

47. The intubation route of choice as suggested by the guidelines for a patient with COPD is

_____

48. Complete the following chart summarizing the ventilator guidelines for COPD patients.

Parameter	Preferred Setting or Range
Tidal volume	_____
Rate	_____
Inspiratory time	_____
Flow rate	_____
Flow waveform	_____
PEEP	_____
F_IO_2	_____

49. Define *pulsus paradoxus*.

_____

_____

_____

50. What are the two main concerns that a respiratory therapist must be aware of during the mechanical ventilation of a patient with acute asthma?

a. _____

b. _____

51. During ventilation of a patient with asthma, plateau pressure should be kept at _____

52. Complete the following chart summarizing the ventilator guidelines for patients with acute severe asthma.

Parameter	Preferred Setting or Range
Tidal volume	_____
Rate	_____
Inspiratory time	_____
Flow rate	_____
Flow waveform	_____
PEEP	_____
F_IO_2	_____

53. Diagnostic percussion during an asthma episode typically reveals _____.

54. List five neuromuscular disorders that may require ventilatory support.

   a. _____

   b. _____

   c. _____

   d. _____

   e. _____

55. What are the main reasons patients with neuromuscular disorders may require ventilatory support?

   _____

   _____

56. Complete the following chart summarizing the ventilator guidelines for patients with neuromuscular disorders.

Parameter	Preferred Setting or Range
Tidal volume	_____
Rate	_____
Inspiratory time	_____
Flow rate	_____
Flow waveform	_____
PEEP	_____
F_IO_2	_____

57. What are the common causes of increased ICPs?

   _____

   _____

   _____

58. As it relates to cerebral perfusion pressure (CPP):
   a. What is the equation for CPP?

   _____

   b. What are the normal values for the components of this formula?

   _____

59. What CPP indicates poor cerebral perfusion?

   _____

60. When and how should iatrogenic hyperventilation be used?

61. Complete the following chart summarizing the ventilator guidelines for patients with closed head injury.

Parameter	Preferred Setting or Range
Tidal volume	_____
Rate	_____
Inspiratory time	_____
Flow rate	_____
Flow waveform	_____
PEEP	_____
F_IO_2	_____

62. List the diagnostic criteria for ARDS.

   a. _____

   b. _____

   c. _____

   d. _____

   e. _____

63. List 10 examples of conditions associated with the development of ARDS.

   a. _____

   b. _____

   c. _____

   d. _____

   e. _____

   f. _____

   g. _____

   h. _____

   i. _____

   j. _____

64. Describe the open lung approach to ventilating patients with ARDS.

   _____

   _____

   _____

65. Complete the following chart summarizing the ventilator guidelines for patients with ARDS.

Parameter	Preferred Setting or Range
Tidal volume	_____
Rate	_____
Inspiratory time	_____
Flow rate	_____
Flow waveform	_____
PEEP	_____
F_IO_2	_____

66. In the management of ARDS, what are the acceptable end points for arterial blood gases?

_____

_____

67. How is refractory hypoxemia identified?

_____

68. How does ARDS present on chest x-ray?

_____

69. A patient with ARDS will have a total lung compliance of less than _____ cm H_2O.

70. The amount of pulmonary shunt that is indicative of ARDS is _____.

71. The pulmonary capillary wedge pressure values that are typically found in patients with ARDS are

_____.

72. Five common causes of acute cardiogenic pulmonary edema and congestive heart failure (CHF) include:

a. _____

b. _____

c. _____

d. _____

e. _____

73. Complete the following chart summarizing the ventilator guidelines for patients with CHF.

Parameter	Preferred Setting or Range
Tidal volume	_____
Rate	_____
Inspiratory time	_____
Flow rate	_____
Flow waveform	_____
PEEP	_____
F_IO_2	_____

74. Patients with CHF and mild to moderate hypoxemia can be successfully managed without intubation using which two modalities?

_____

CRITICAL THINKING QUESTIONS

1. Discuss the pros and cons for using sighs with mechanical ventilation.

_____

_____

_____

_____

_____

_____

2. Explain the progression of an asthma episode from arrival to the emergency department to intubation and mechanical ventilation.

_____

_____

_____

_____

_____

_____

_____

_____

3. Discuss why the use of pressure-support ventilation (PSV) may not be appropriate for patients with COPD.

_____

_____

_____

_____

_____

_____

4. Why is it important for expiratory time to be maximized when ventilating a patient with increased airway resistance, such as with asthma or COPD?

_____

_____

_____

CASE STUDIES

Case Study 1

A 62-year-old male weighs 256 pounds and is 73 inches tall. The patient has a history of congestive heart failure and has been placed on a nonrebreathing mask at 15 L/min. Physical assessment reveals the patient is alert and oriented but anxious and diaphoretic. Vital signs are as follows: pulse 142 beats/min and thready, blood pressure 105/68 mm Hg, oral temperature 98.6°F, and respiratory rate 26 breaths/min shallow and labored. Breath sounds reveal bilateral inspiratory coarse crackles. The arterial blood gas on the nonrebreathing mask is pH 7.24, P_aCO_2 51 mm Hg, P_aO_2 42 mm Hg, and HCO_3^- 23 mEq/L. The patient's electrocardiogram shows a widened QRS complex with occasional premature ventricular contractions.

1. What respiratory care intervention is indicated at this time?

_____

_____

2. If this patient is intubated and placed on mechanical ventilation, what mode, tidal volume, and rate would you suggest?

_____

_____

Case Study 2

A motor vehicle crash victim arrives at the hospital via ambulance. The 37-year-old patient has sustained a closed head injury. Physical assessment reveals a pulse of 145 beats/min, respiratory rate 32 breaths/min, and blood pressure 155/97 mm Hg. Her neck veins are distended, and she is diaphoretic. She is 68 inches tall and weighs 175 pounds. The patient has no history of cardiac or respiratory disease. The patient has an oral airway in place with a weak gag reflex. On 60% oxygen, the arterial blood gas is pH 7.22, P_aCO_2 64 mm Hg, P_aO_2 78 mm Hg, S_aO_2 92%, and HCO_3^- 25 mEq/L.

1. What type of respiratory failure appears to be present in this patient?

_____

_____

2. What acid-base imbalance is present?

_____

3. What type of mechanical ventilatory support may this patient benefit from?

_____

4. What are the appropriate parameters for this patient, including minute ventilation, tidal volume, inspiratory time, flow rate, and PEEP?

_____

_____

_____

Case Study 3

A 40-year-old female, height 66 inches and weight 156 pounds, presents to the emergency department with the chief complaint of shortness of breath. She is alert, very anxious, unable to complete a sentence without stopping to take a breath, and is sitting in a tripod position. Her heart rate is 136 beats/min and regular; respirations are 30 breaths/min and very labored with accessory muscle use. Her blood pressure is 168/84 mm Hg, and her oral temperature is 37.2°C. Breath sounds are decreased bilaterally with expiratory wheezes. She has a weak, nonproductive cough. The patient has been receiving continuous aerosol albuterol and has received intravenous Solu-Medrol. The patient's best peak flow after bronchodilator therapy is 150 L/min with her normal best typically around 500 L/min. Arterial blood gas results while on nasal cannula 6 L/min show pH 7.34, P_aCO_2 42 mm Hg, P_aO_2 48 mm Hg, S_aO_2 79%, and HCO_3^- 22 mEq/L.

1. How should this blood gas be interpreted?

_____

_____

_____

2. Does the situation warrant intubation and mechanical ventilation? Why or why not?

_____

_____

_____

3. What type of mechanical ventilatory support may this patient benefit from?

_____

_____

4. If pressure-controlled (PC)-CMV is used for this patient, what are the appropriate settings (including PIP setting, resulting tidal volume, respiratory rate, inspiratory time, waveform, and PEEP)?

_____

_____

_____

Case Study 4

A 64-year-old, 197-pound, 6-foot 1-inch male patient was admitted 3 days ago for a COPD exacerbation. He is currently receiving supplemental oxygen via nasal cannula at 3 L/min, albuterol and ipratropium every 4 hours, and an intravenous corticosteroid and antibiotic. He has bilaterally diminished breath sounds with rhonchi in both bases with a weak, nonproductive cough. A chest x-ray from this morning shows bibasilar infiltrates. The current arterial blood gas results reveal pH 7.32, P_aCO_2 57 mm Hg, P_aO_2 54 mm Hg, S_aO_2 85%, and HCO_3^- 29 mEq/L.

1. How should this blood gas be interpreted?

_____

2. Does the situation warrant intubation and mechanical ventilation? Why or why not?

_____

_____

_____

3. If intubation is required what mode and parameters would you suggest for this patient?

_____

_____

NBRC-STYLE QUESTIONS

1. Which of the following is (are) true concerning the use of permissive hypercapnia in the management of ARDS?
   1. Keep $P_{plateau}$ below 30 cm H_2O by lowering V_T to 4 to 6 mL/kg.
   2. P_aCO_2 should go no higher than 60 mm Hg.
   3. High $PEEP_E$ levels greater than 15 cm H_2O may be required.
   4. The P_aCO_2 is permitted to rise rapidly to the acceptable level.
   a. 1 and 3 only
   b. 2 and 4 only
   c. 1 and 4 only
   d. 2 and 3 only

2. A mechanically ventilated patient has been using an HME for humidification for the past 72 hours. During rounds and chart review, the respiratory therapist notices a steady increase in PIP over the past 2 days. The respiratory therapist suctions the patient to assess the secretions. The secretions are very thick and tenacious. The most appropriate action at this time is which of the following?
   a. Suction the patient more often.
   b. Add a passover humidifier to the system.
   c. Switch to a heated wick-type humidifier.
   d. Use normal saline to lavage before suctioning.

3. A 75-year-old female, admitted through the emergency department earlier today, is increasingly distressed and unable to breathe comfortably except in the upright position. She has a history of coronary artery disease, and on admission, she was complaining of chest pain. She is becoming increasingly short of breath and appears cyanotic. Vital signs reveal pulse 142 beats/min, blood pressure 150/92 mm Hg, and respiratory rate 30 breaths/min and labored. The arterial blood gas on nasal cannula 3 L/min is pH 7.18, P_aCO_2 81 mm Hg, P_aO_2 35 mm Hg, S_aO_2 79%, and HCO_3^- 29 mEq/L. The respiratory therapist should recommendation which of the following?
   a. Nasal mask CPAP at +10 cm H_2O
   b. Nonrebreathing mask with 15 L/min oxygen
   c. Bilevel PAP: Inspiratory positive airway pressure (IPAP) 15 cm H2O and expiratory positive airway pressure (EPAP) 5 cm H_2O
   d. Intubation and mechanical ventilation with PC-CMV

4. Appropriate ventilatory parameters for an otherwise healthy 185-pound, 6-foot 1-inch, 26-year-old male patient who was brought to the emergency department because of a drug overdose include which of the following?
   a. VC-CMV, tidal volume 600 mL, set rate 12 breaths/min
   b. VC-IMV, tidal volume 600 mL, set rate 6 breaths/min
   c. PC-CMV, set pressure 25 cm H_2O, inspiratory time 1.5 seconds
   d. Pressure support ventilation of 15 cm H_2O with CPAP 5 cm H_2O.

5. Before intubation, a patient's P_aO_2 was 78 mm Hg while receiving an F_IO_2 of 0.60. What F_IO_2 setting on the ventilator will bring the P_aO_2 up to 90 mm Hg? (Assume that this patient's cardiopulmonary status and respiratory quotient are constant.)
   a. 0.70
   b. 0.75
   c. 0.80
   d. 0.85

6. A patient has just been intubated in the emergency department. The patient is a 64-year-old obese male patient with a suspected drug overdose. The patient is 6 feet tall and weighs 435 pounds. The most appropriate tidal volume to ventilate this patient is which of the following?
   a. 380 mL
   b. 640 mL
   c. 810 mL
   d. 975 mL

7. Which of the following ventilatory parameters is appropriate when mechanically ventilating a patient with COPD?
   a. Use a rectangle flow waveform.
   b. Set tidal volume between 10 and 15 mL/kg.
   c. Use peak inspiratory flow rates greater than 60 L/min.
   d. Institute PEEP in the range of 5 to 10 cm H_2O.

8. A patient with ARDS has been changed from VC-CMV to PC-CMV. When this change was made, there was an increase in mean airway pressure. Which of the following statements is true concerning elevated mean airway pressures?
   a. The mean airway pressure increases with longer expiratory times.
   b. An increased mean airway pressure may result in improved oxygenation.
   c. Elevated mean airway pressures decrease the risk of barotraumas.
   d. High mean airway pressures increase the risk of cardiovascular side effects.

9. A 5-feet 4-inches tall, 125-pound female patient who has just been intubated because of a severe asthma episode would be ventilated most appropriately with which of the following ventilator parameters?
   a. PSV 20 cm H_2O with CPAP +10 cm H_2O
   b. PC-CMV, 12 breath/min, PIP 25 cm H_2O, T_I 0.75 second
   c. VC-IMV, 12 breath/min, V_T 800 mL, flow 50 L/min, rectangle waveform
   d. VC-CMV, 10 breath/min, V_T 570 mL, flow 35 L/min, descending waveform

10. HMEs may not be appropriate for use with infants, children, and small adults due to which of the following?
    a. Presence of mechanical dead space in the HMEs
    b. Increased rate of endotracheal occlusion with these patients
    c. Patients' inability to overcome resistance across the HME
    d. HMEs inability to provide adequate humidity for these patients

HELPFUL INTERNET SITES:

- N.S. Ward, K.M. Dushay, "Clinical Concise Review: Mechanical Ventilation of Patients with Chronic Obstructive Pulmonary Disease," *Crit Care Med* (2008): 36(5):1614-619.
  http://www.ncbi.nlm.nih.gov/pubmed/18434881
- A.A. Sovari, "Cardiogenic Pulmonary Edema" *Medscape Reference*.
  http://emedicine.medscape.com/article/157452-overview
- ARDSNet: NIH NHLBI ARDS Clinical, Network Mechanical Ventilation Protocol Summary, search for "Mechanical Ventilation Protocol Summary" http://www.ardsnet.org/

Initial Patient Assessment

LEARNING OBJECTIVES

Upon completion of this chapter, the reader will be able to do the following:

1. Understand the importance of performing an operational verification procedure.
2. State the recommended times when an oxygen analyzer is used to measure the fractional inspired oxygen concentration (F_IO_2) during mechanical ventilation.
3. Identify various pathophysiologic conditions that alter a patient's transairway pressure, peak pressure, and plateau pressure.
4. Use pressure-time and flow-time curves obtained during pressure-controlled continuous mandatory ventilation to determine the plateau pressure.
5. Identify a system leak from a volume-time curve.
6. Use physical examination and radiographic data to determine whether pneumonia, acute respiratory distress syndrome (ARDS), flail chest, pneumothorax, asthma, pleural effusion, or emphysema is present.
7. Determine whether a lung compliance problem or an airway resistance problem is present using the ventilator flow sheet and time, volume, peak inspiratory pressure (PIP), and plateau pressure data.
8. Evaluate a static pressure-volume curve for static compliance and dynamic compliance to determine changes in compliance or resistance.
9. Estimate a patient's alveolar ventilation based on ideal body weight, tidal volume, and respiratory rate.
10. Detect a cuff leak by listening to breath sounds.
11. Recognize inappropriate endotracheal tube cuff pressures and an inappropriate tube size and recommend measures to correct these problems.
12. Evaluate flow sheet information about a patient on pressure control ventilation and recommend methods for determining whether compliance and airway resistance have changed.
13. Explain the technique for measuring endotracheal tube cuff pressure using a manometer, syringe, and three-way stopcock.
14. Describe two methods that can be used to remedy a cut pilot tube (pilot balloon line) without changing the endotracheal tube.

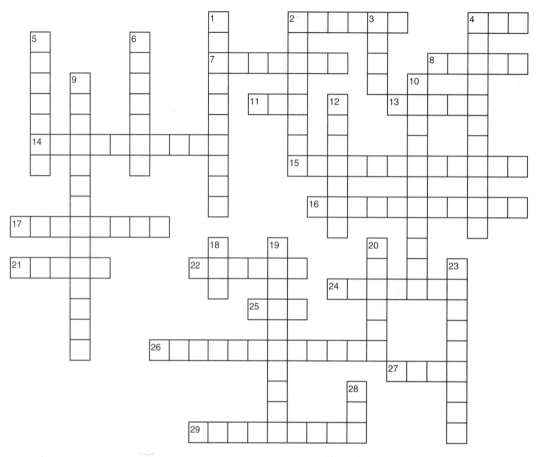

Across

2 A place to measure temperature
4 Something in the ventilator circuit that adds dead space (abbreviation)
7 A cause of abdominal distention due to fluid
8 The _____ inflection point indicates a time at which large numbers of alveoli are becoming overinflated
11 A multipart procedure to check that a ventilator is working properly (abbreviation)
13 A cuffed endotracheal tube has a _____ balloon
14 A common place for leaks
15 It puts air in the pleural space and reduces lung compliance
16 The setting that allows patient triggering
17 Cell death
21 The _____ inflection point indicates the pressure at which large numbers of alveoli are being recruited
22 Type of compliance measured at no flow
24 Type of compliance that is measured during gas movement
25 A pressure that can be measured continuously by a flow-directed catheter (abbreviation)
26 Another term used to describe tubing compliance is _____ volume
27 Another name for base flow is _____ flow
29 The form on which the patient-ventilator check is written (two words)

Down

1 Type of pressure that is important to tissue oxygenation and affects both lung volumes and cardiac output (two words)
2 Dynamic hyperinflation (two words)
3 When exhaled tidal volume is less than set tidal volume there is a _____
4 A condition of low body temperature
5 A breath sound that indicates the possible need for suctioning
6 A type of recoil
9 It puts fluid in the alveoli and reduces lung compliance (two words)
10 A place where the central venous pressure catheter dwells (two words)
12 A breath sound that indicates the possible need for bronchodilator therapy
18 The amount of pressure needed to overcome airway resistance (abbreviation)
19 Heart rate, respiratory rate, and blood pressure are all part of this (two words)
20 Tidal volume multiplied by respiratory rate (frequency) equals _____ ventilation
23 The secondary respiratory muscles
28 Method for ensuring no leaks around an endotracheal tube (abbreviation)

Chapter 8 Initial Patient Assessment

CHAPTER REVIEW QUESTIONS

1. List eight observations that the clinician should make when assessing the physiologic status of a patient receiving mechanical ventilation.

   a. _____

   b. _____

   c. _____

   d. _____

   e. _____

   f. _____

   g. _____

   h. _____

2. Documentation of patient information and ventilator settings should be made on the _____ .

3. Before a ventilator can be used on a patient, the respiratory therapist must confirm this procedure was performed and passed on that ventilator.

   _____

4. In addition to regularly timed checks, list six instances when patient-ventilator system checks should be performed.

   a. _____

   b. _____

   c. _____

   d. _____

   e. _____

   f. _____

5. If continuous F_IO_2 measurement is not available on a particular ventilator, how often should it be measured for:

   a. An adult? _____

   b. An infant?_____

6. What is the first thing the clinician should assess following a patient being connected to a mechanical ventilator? _____

7. How long should a clinician wait after the initiation of mechanical ventilation to draw an arterial blood gas sample?

   _____

8. The appropriate range for pressure-trigger setting (sensitivity setting) is

   _____

9. The appropriate range for flow triggering setting (sensitivity setting) is

   _____

10. a. How does auto-PEEP make triggering the ventilator more difficult for a patient?

    b. How can triggering the ventilator be made easier without causing autotriggering?

    a. _____

    b. _____

11. Describe a strategy may be used to eliminate or reduce auto-PEEP.

    _____

    _____

    _____

    _____

12. What effect would a heat moisture exchanger attached to the endotracheal tube have on alveolar ventilation?

    _____

    _____

13. Calculate the alveolar minute ventilation if the set V_T is 775 mL, ideal body weight is 160 pounds, and added V_D is 85 mL.

    _____

    _____

14. List two factors to consider when determining alveolar ventilation.

    a. _____

    b. _____

15. An increase in PIP is likely due to a _____ in compliance or an _____ in airway resistance.

16. What ventilator maneuver must be performed to measure plateau pressure?

    _____

17. Describe a clinical scenario that would result in an inaccurate plateau pressure measurement.

_____

_____

18. Ideally, a plateau pressure should be kept below _____ to avoid lung injury.

19. What pressure measurements are needed to calculate dynamic compliance?

_____

20. What pressure measurements are needed to calculate static compliance?

_____

21. Define *transairway pressure.*

_____

_____

22. What does an increase in the difference between PIP and $P_{plateau}$ indicate?

_____

_____

23. List four possible causes for increased airway resistance in a patient on mechanical ventilation.

a. _____

b. _____

c. _____

d. _____

24. What is the significance of monitoring mean airway pressure?

_____

_____

25. What maneuver is performed to assess auto-PEEP?

_____

26. The high pressure limit alarm is usually set at about _____ cm H_2O above the measured PIP, and when activated it will _____.

27. List four possible causes that would activate the high pressure limit alarm.

a. _____

b. _____

c. _____

d. _____

28. The low pressure alarm is usually set about _____ cm H_2O below the measured PIP, and when activated usually indicates _____.

29. What is a common cause of activation of the low pressure alarm?

_____

30. If the leak is not obvious, what should you do while you further investigate the source? _____

31. What are two methods the clinician can use to determine whether a leak is present?

a. _____

b. _____

32. If a leak is present, what steps should be taken to find the source?

_____

_____

_____

_____

33. What effect would a leak have during pressure-support ventilation?

_____

34. Describe the following techniques used to inflate tube cuffs:

a. Minimum occlusion technique: _____

b. Minimum leak technique: _____

35. List the factors that can cause hyperthermia.

_____

_____

_____

36. The central venous pressure (CVP) directly reflects what pressures?

_____

_____

37. At what point during a ventilator breath should the CVP measurement be taken?

_____

38. Describe a clinical scenario where a patient would benefit from the monitoring of their pulmonary artery pressure.

_____

_____

39. How often should a physical examination of a ventilated patient be performed?

_____

40. What should be included in the physical examination?

_____

41. Describe the effect abdominal distention has on ventilation.

_____

42. Endotracheal or tracheostomy cuff pressure should be maintained in what range?

_____

43. Describe a clinical scenario where a cuff pressure of 25 mm Hg could cause tracheal damage.

_____

44. List the five-step protocol designed to minimize the risk of tracheal necrosis associated with endotracheal tube cuff overinflation.

a. _____

b. _____

c. _____

d. _____

e. _____

45. List two situations in which a higher-than-acceptable cuff pressure may be required to maintain a minimal occlusion?

a. _____

b. _____

46. Describe the procedure for maintaining cuff pressure if the pilot balloon is accidentally cut.

_____

_____

47. Why should an endotracheal tube be repositioned?

_____

48. The normal value for static compliance (C_S) is

_____.

49. The formula for C_S is

_____.

50. List eight possible causes for a decrease in C_S.

a. _____

b. _____

c. _____

d. _____

e. _____

f. _____

g. _____

h. _____

51. During pressure ventilation, if the set inspiratory pressure remains constant, what effect would a decreased C_S have on tidal volume (V_T)?

_____

52. What is dynamic compliance (C_D)?

_____.

53. C_D decreases whenever C_S _____ or R_{aw} _____.

69

54. During volume ventilation what effect would a decrease in C_D have on PIP and the delivered V_T?

_____

_____

_____

55. Calculate the C_S when the V_T is 740 mL, $P_{plateau}$ is 44 cm H_2O, and the end-expiratory pressure is +8 cm H_2O.

_____

_____

56. Calculate the R_{aw} when the PIP is 58 cm H_2O, $P_{plateau}$ is 51 cm H_2O, and the flow is 0.5 L/s.

_____

_____

_____

57. Identify the problem in Figure 8-1.

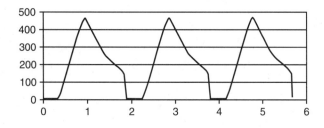

_____

58. What is the plateau pressure in Figure 8-2?

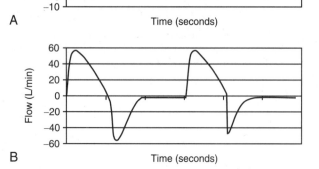

A

Time (seconds)

B

Time (seconds)

_____

59. Calculate the static compliance for the information in Figure 8-2 using the returned tidal volume of 450 mL.

_____

CRITICAL THINKING QUESTIONS

1. During a patient-ventilator system check the clinician notices the patient making inspiratory efforts (patient is using accessory muscles), but the ventilator is not triggering. What could be causing the problem? What steps could be taken to correct it?

_____

_____

_____

2. A 250-pound adult male has a 6.5-mm inner diameter endotracheal tube in place and is being mechanically ventilated. Cuff pressures of 40 cm H_2O are required to maintain an adequate seal. What recommendations should be made to correct this problem?

_____

_____

_____

3. A patient with ARDS is being managed on pressure-controlled ventilation, with a set inspiratory pressure of 30 cm H_2O. According to the ventilator flow sheet, measured tidal volumes for the past 3 days have ranged between 400 and 450 mL. During the first ventilator-patient system check of the day, the respiratory therapist notes that the measured tidal volume is now 550 mL, without any change in the set pressure parameters. What is likely the cause of the tidal volume increase?

_____

_____

_____

4. When the PIP is 43 cm H_2O and the plateau pressure is 18 cm H_2O, how much pressure is required to overcome the resistance of the airways?

_____

Case Study 1

A respiratory therapist is called to a code in the intensive care unit (ICU). After the patient is stabilized, the physician writes the following order for mechanical ventilation: volume control, V_T 700 mL, f 12, F_IO_2 1.0, PEEP +5 cm H_2O. The respiratory therapist observes a PIP of 42 cm H_2O with the order settings.

1. At what levels should the high- and low-pressure alarms be set?

    _____

    _____

2. At what level should the low V_T alarm be set?

    _____

3. How would the respiratory therapist obtain a plateau pressure?

    _____

4. What should the therapist recommend if the plateau pressure measurement obtained was 38 cm H_2O?

    _____

    _____

    _____

Case Study 2

An obtunded patient in the ICU has been receiving volume ventilation CV-CMV for the past 3 days. Today the patient appears to be responsive and wakening up. The high-pressure, low-minute volume, and low tidal volume alarms are activating frequently, and the patient appears to be agitated and confused.

1. Indicate possible causes for the high-pressure alarm activating.

    _____

    _____

2. What could be a cause for the low-minute volume and low tidal volume alarms being activated?

    _____

    _____

3. What recommendations would you make to resolve the problem?

    _____

    _____

Case Study 3

A 38-year-old female patient was admitted through the emergency department 24 hours ago following a motor vehicle crash. She was intubated in the field due to respiratory arrest secondary to blunt chest trauma. She also sustained four fractured ribs. The patient is currently on VC-CMV, f 15 breath/min, V_T 440 mL, F_IO_2 0.8, PEEP +8 cm H_2O. The following values were obtained on those ventilator settings.

Time	PIP (cm H_2O)	$P_{plateau}$ (cm H_2O)	Exhaled V_T (mL)
0800	35	30	440
1000	39	34	440
1100	45	39	440
1130	50	44	440

1. What is the P_{ta} for each patient-ventilator system check?

    _____

2. What is the likely cause for the increasing PIP over the course of the 3.5 hours?

    _____

    _____

    _____

3. What are some of the most likely causes of this problem?

    _____

    _____

4. How would you assess the patient to determine the appropriate treatment?

    _____

    _____

    _____

Case Study 4

A 56-year-old male patient with a history of COPD was admitted yesterday with a diagnosis of pneumonia. During the night he was intubated due to respiratory arrest. The patient is currently receiving VC-CMV, f 12 breath/min, V_T 525 mL, F_IO_2 0.4, PEEP +3 cm H_2O. The following values were obtained on those ventilator settings.

Time	PIP (cm H_2O)	$P_{plateau}$ (cm H_2O)	Exhaled V_T (mL)
0630	36	23	525
0835	39	22	523
1030	41	23	525
1230	46	19	524

1. What is the P_{ta} for each patient-ventilator system check?

_____

2. What is the likely cause for the increasing PIP over the course of the 6 hours?

_____

_____

_____

3. What are some of the most likely causes of this problem?

_____

_____

4. How would you assess and treat this patient?

_____

_____

_____

NBRC-STYLE QUESTIONS

1. An increase in the peak inspiratory flow rate would increase which of the following?
   a. Tidal volume
   b. Total cycle time
   c. Expiratory time
   d. Inspiratory time

2. A patient receiving volume-controlled mechanical ventilation has a decrease in static compliance. Which of the following would most likely occur?
   a. An increase in tidal volume
   b. A decrease in minute ventilation
   c. An increase in PIP
   d. An increased inspiratory-to-expiratory ratio

3. While monitoring endotracheal cuff pressures during a patient-ventilator system check, the therapist obtains a reading of 44 cm H_2O. What should the therapist do next?
   a. Get a syringe and add air to the cuff.
   b. Insert a smaller diameter endotracheal tube.
   c. No changes need to be made; the cuff pressure is acceptable.
   d. Release air from the cuff until minimal occluding volume is achieved.

4. Which of the following can cause a mechanically ventilated patient's PIP to increase from 20 to 40 cm H_2O rapidly while the static compliance remains relatively unchanged?
   a. Recently removal of mucous plugs
   b. Decreased airway resistance
   c. Tension pneumothorax
   d. Decreased elastance

5. Which of the following can cause an increase in PIP and plateau pressure with a stable transairway pressure?
   a. ARDS
   b. Acute asthma exacerbation
   c. Retained secretions in the airways
   d. An endotracheal tube that is too small

6. While responding to a ventilator alarm, the respiratory therapist sees that the low-pressure alarm is activated. She hears an audible leak, and notices that the exhaled volume is 200 mL below the set tidal volume. The measured cuff pressure is 15 mm Hg. What action should be taken next?
   a. Replace the endotracheal tube with a larger size.
   b. Increase the patient's V_T to compensate for the leak.
   c. Introduce enough volume into the cuff to maintain a pressure of less than 20 cm H_2O.
   d. While auscultating the larynx, introduce enough air into the cuff until a slight leak is heard on peak inspiration.

7. Why is positive end-expiratory pressure (PEEP) subtracted from plateau pressure when calculating C_s?
   a. To compensate for a loss in volume due to a leak
   b. To determine auto-PEEP
   c. To determine the actual pressure change
   d. To calculate the actual PEEP level

8. Which of the following may cause an increase in heart rate?
   1. Hypoxemia
   2. Hypothermia
   3. Anxiety
   4. Pain
   a. 1 only
   b. 1 and 3 only
   c. 1, 2, and 3 only
   d. 1, 3, and 4 only

9. Which of the following physical findings would you expect when assessing an asthmatic patient?
   1. Late inspiratory crackles
   2. Hyper-resonant percussion note
   3. Accessory muscle use
   4. Tracheal shift
   a. 1 only
   b. 1 and 3 only
   c. 2 and 3 only
   d. 2, 3, and 4 only

10. Evaluate the following data from the patient's flow sheet.

Time	Set V_T	PIP (cm H_2O)	$P_{plateau}$ (cm H_2O)
4:00	700 mL	38	32
5:00	700 mL	41	34
6:00	700 mL	47	32

Based on the above data which of the following statements is true?
   a. C_L is improving.
   b. There is no change in C_L.
   c. R_{aw} is improving.
   d. There is an increase in R_{aw}.

9 Ventilator Graphics

Upon completion of this chapter, the reader will be able to do the following:

1. Identify ventilator variables (e.g., the target variable and trigger variable) and ventilator parameters and their values (e.g., peak inspiratory pressure [PIP] and plateau pressure) using pressure, flow, and volume scalars generated using various modes of mechanical ventilation.

2. Identify ventilator variables and ventilator parameters and their values from flow-volume and pressure-volume loops.

3. Use ventilator scalars and loops to detect changes in lung compliance and airway resistance, inappropriate sensitivity settings, inadequate inspiratory flow, auto-PEEP, leaks in the ventilator circuit, active exhalation during pressure-support ventilation (PSV), and an inspiratory pressure overshoot during PSV.

4. Calculate airway resistance and lung compliance using values derived from scalars and loops generated during mechanical ventilation.

5. Explain the changes that occur in scalars and loops during volume-targeted and pressure-targeted ventilation when airway resistance increases and lung compliances decreases.

6. Given a compliance value obtained during pressure-controlled ventilation (PCV), determine tidal volume delivery, and recommend ways to adjust the set pressure to gain a desired tidal volume.

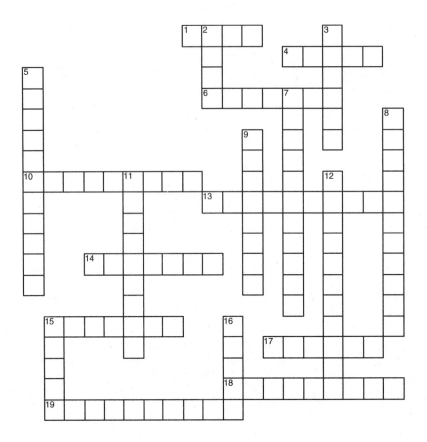

Across

1 Volume per unit of time
4 This control adjusts the rate at which the flow valve opens
6 Pressure reading when inspiration is held
10 Easy to inflate
13 The difference between the inspiratory and expiratory curves in a pressure-volume loop
14 Begins inspiration
15 A way to specify the waveforms for pressure, flow, and volume that are graphed against time
17 One variable plotted against time
18 Matching of the onset of breath by the ventilator and patient effort
19 The frictional forces associated with ventilation

Down

2 Two variables, other than time, plotted against each other
3 Flow multiplied by inspiratory time
5 When patient and ventilator are not working together
7 Rapid rise or decay on a graph
8 Name of pressure gradient required to overcome airway resistance
9 Type of flow that creates a wave form parallel to the x-axis
11 Type of positive end-expiratory pressure (PEEP) caused by air trapping
12 A square wave is also known as _____
15 Adjusting the rise of pressure or flow to the patient
16 This is necessary to measure plateau pressure

CHAPTER REVIEW QUESTIONS

1. Identify the scalar shapes in Figure 9-1.

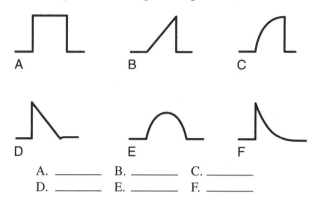

A   B   C

D   E   F

A. _____ B. _____ C. _____
D. _____ E. _____ F. _____

2. What is the difference between a scalar and a loop?

_____

3. What is the mathematical relationship between volume, flow, and inspiratory time?

_____

4. List the two factors that determine the flow of gas into the lungs.

a. _____

b. _____

5. As lung compliance increases, the pressure required to deliver the volume to the patient is _____. When lung compliance decreases, the pressure required to deliver the volume to the patient is _____.

6. The pressure at the mouth (P_{awo}) is equal to the sum of what two pressures?

_____

7. When does the flow-time curve run parallel to the x-axis?

_____

8. Calculate the T_I in seconds when the volume is 600 mL and the flow rate is 60 L/min.

_____

9. Calculate P_A when the delivered volume is 800 mL and static compliance is 25 mL/cm H_2O.

_____

10. Identify the labeled parts of the flow-time scalar in Figure 9-2.

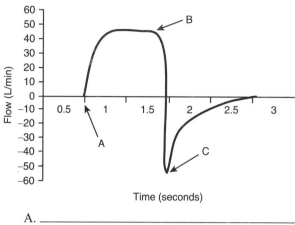

Time (seconds)

A. _____

B. _____

C. _____

For Questions 11 through 14, refer to the flow waveform in Figure 9-3.

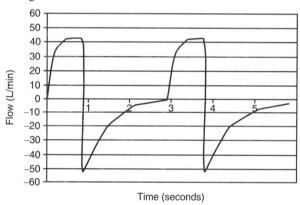

Time (seconds)

11. What type of flow waveform is shown in the figure?

_____

12. What is the peak inspiratory flow rate?

_____

13. What is the peak expiratory flow rate?

_____

14. What is the approximate inspiratory time? _____

_____

15. What is the expiratory time? _____

16. You have a patient with an exacerbation of asthma who was just intubated. The chest radiograph reveals a flattened diaphragm. What is the likely cause for the flow curve not returning to zero at the end of exhalation?

_____

17. Your patient was coughing when you attempted an inspiratory hold maneuver. Would the measurement be accurate? Why or why not?

_____

18. At what point in the breath cycle does the intrinsic PEEP measurement occur?

_____

19. In Figure 9-4, what is the reason for the increase in flow (*point A*) at the end of inspiration?

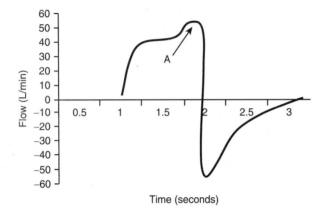

Time (seconds)

_____

20. What is the appropriate initial pressure trigger setting for an adult patient? _____

21. Asynchrony between the patient and the ventilator may be caused by inappropriate settings of which two parameters?

_____

22. How does changing the flow pattern affect PIP during volume ventilation?

_____

For Questions 23 through 29, refer to the pressure, volume, and flow curves for VC-CMV in the graphs in Figure 9-5.

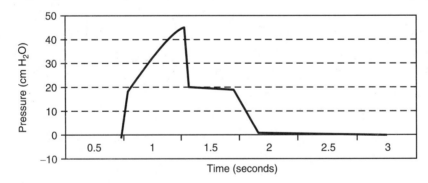

Time (seconds)

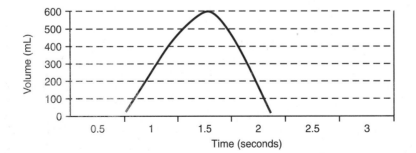

Time (seconds)

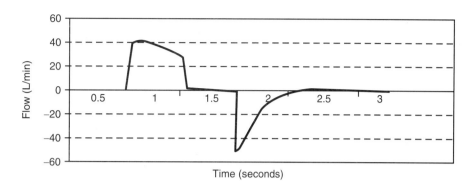

23. What is the PIP? _____

24. What is the set flow pattern and rate? _____

25. What is the tidal volume? _____

26. Calculate the static compliance.

    _____

27. Calculate the airway resistance.

    _____

28. Is intrinsic PEEP present? _____

29. Why does the flow rate drop to zero before the end of inspiration?

    _____

30. During PCV, the patient's lung compliance drops. How will this affect the delivered volume?

    _____

31. During PC-CMV, why does flow return to zero before the end of inspiration?

    _____

32. What type of flow waveform is used during PCV?

    _____

33. When does the highest pressure gradient between the ventilator and the lungs occur?

    _____

34. What parameters need to be set to deliver PSV?

    _____

35. Identify the ventilator mode from Figure 9-6.

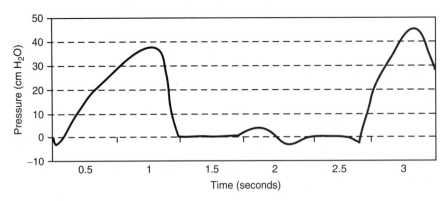

For Questions 36 and 37, refer to Figure 9-7.

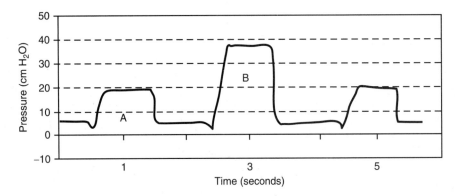

36. Identify the mode of ventilation. _____

37. Identify waves *A* and *B*. _____

38. Explain how automatic tube compensation works on inspiration and expiration.

_____

39. If the peak flow rate for a pressure support breath is 45 L/min and the flow cycle percent is set at 25%, at what flow rate will inspiration end?

_____

For Questions 40 through 44, refer to the flow curve for a PSV breath in Figure 9-8.

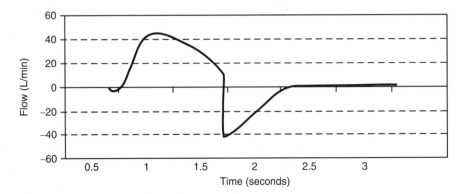

40. What is the T$_I$ for this breath? _____

41. What is the peak inspiratory flow rate for this breath? _____

42. At what flow rate did inspiration end? _____

43. What is the flow cycle percent setting? _____

44. What is the peak expiratory flow rate? _____

45. Explain why a patient with chronic obstructive pulmonary disease (COPD) requires a higher flow cycle percent for PS breaths.

   _____

46. Explain why a patient with stiff lungs gains the most benefit during PSV with a low flow cycle percent setting.

   _____

For Questions 47 through 52, refer to the flow, pressure, and volume scalars represented in Figure 9-9. The scalars labeled *A* are the flow, pressure, and volume scalars for a single ventilator breath. The scalars labeled *B* refer to a second ventilator breath.

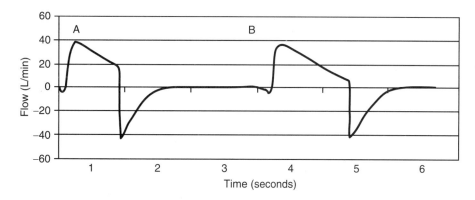

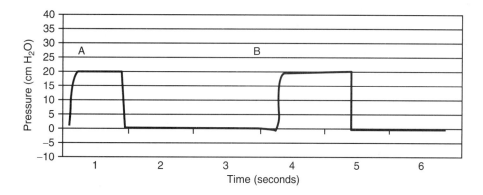

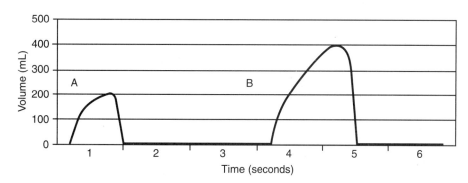

47. What is the approximate flow cycle percent in *A*?

_____

48. What is the patient tidal volume in *A*?

_____

49. What is the approximate flow cycle percent in *B*?

_____

50. What is the patient tidal volume in *B*? _____

51. What are the approximate inspiratory times in breaths *A* and *B*?

_____

52. Why is the T_I longer for *B* than for *A*? _____

For Questions 53 through 56, refer to the pressure-volume loop in Figure 9-10.

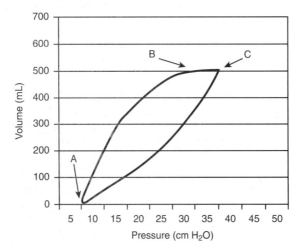

53. Identify points *A*, *B*, and *C*.

_____

54. What is the PIP?

_____

55. What is the tidal volume?

_____

56. Why does the loop begin and end at 5 cm H_2O?

_____

57. What happens to a pressure-volume loop when lung compliance decreases during VC-CMV?

_____

58. What happens to a pressure-volume loop when lung compliance decreases during PC-CMV?

_____

59. What causes the pressure-volume loop to widen or bulge?

_____

For Questions 60 through 65, refer to the pressure-volume loops in Figure 9-11.

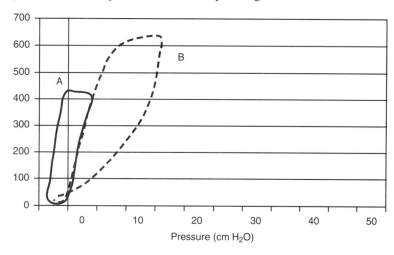

60. What type of breath does loop *A* represent?

_____

61. In which direction does loop *A* move? Why?

_____

62. What type of breath does loop *B* represent?

_____

63. In which direction does loop *B* move? Why?

_____

64. The set flow is 45 L/min; calculate the R_{aw}.

_____

65. The difference between the inspiratory and expiratory curves on a volume-pressure loop is called

_____

For Questions 66 through 69, refer to the flow-volume loop in Figure 9-12.

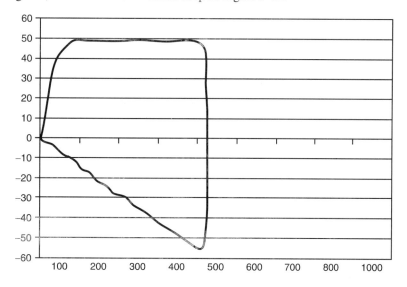

Chapter **9** **Ventilator Graphics**

66. In which direction does this loop move?

_____

67. What type of flow waveform is represented?

_____

68. The set inspiratory flow rate is _____, and the peak expiratory flow rate is

_____

69. What is the tidal volume?

_____

70. What can cause the expiratory side of a flow-volume loop to end at a volume above zero?

_____

71. What can cause a gap between the inspiratory side and expiratory side on the zero intercept of the *y*-axis (flow) of a flow-volume loop?

_____

CRITICAL THINKING QUESTIONS

For Questions 1 through 8, refer to the graphs in Figure 9-13.

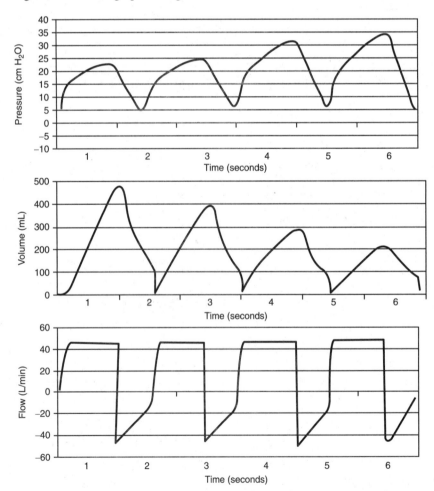

1. What mode of ventilation is being delivered?

   _____

2. Is this patient assisting?

   _____

3. What are the total cycle time, T_I, expiratory time, and set rate?

   _____

   _____

4. Describe the problem that is noticeable on the pressure-time curve.

   _____

5. Describe the two problems that are noticeable on the volume-time curve.

   _____

   _____

6. Describe the problem that is noticeable on the flow-time curve.

   _____

   _____

   _____

7. Taking into consideration the three scalars, what is causing these waveform problems?

   _____

   _____

   _____

   _____

8. What can be done to eliminate the cause of these problems?

   _____

   _____

CASE STUDIES

Case Study 1

A 68-year-old female who is 6 feet tall and weighs 120 lb was admitted through the emergency department with crushing chest pain. The patient has a history of COPD. Cardiac angiography was performed, and the patient subsequently underwent coronary artery bypass surgery. She now is in the cardiovascular intensive care unit (ICU) receiving mechanical ventilation. Figure 9-14 shows a current pressure-volume loop for this patient.

1. What accounts for the shape of this loop?

   _____

   _____

   _____

   _____

2. Is the patient triggering the ventilator? Explain.

   _____

   _____

   _____

3. What is the set tidal volume?

   _____

   _____

   _____

   _____

4. What is the PIP? _____

5. How should the ventilator settings be changed at this time?

_____

_____

_____

_____

_____

Case Study 2

You are the respiratory therapist in the ICU of a large municipal hospital. During rounds you note the pressure-volume loop in Figure 9-15 for one of your patients.

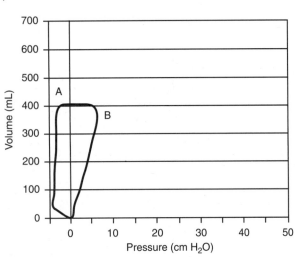

1. What type of breath is represented?

_____

2. What does the portion of the loop labeled *A* represent?

_____

3. What does the portion of the loop labeled *B* represent?

_____

4. This type of loop moves in what direction?

_____

5. Has PS been set for this patient? Explain.

_____

_____

_____

At the next patient-ventilator system check for this individual, you note the pressure-volume loop shown in Figure 9-16.

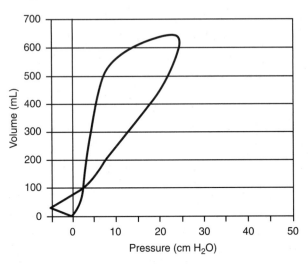

6. What type of ventilatory support is the patient receiving?

_____

7. Is the patient making some inspiratory effort?

_____

8. What ventilator adjustment is most appropriate for this patient at this time? Why?

_____

_____

You change the graphic display and now see the graph shown in Figure 9-17.

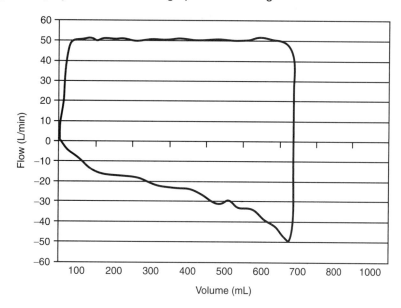

9. What data can be obtained from this loop?

_____

_____

An hour later, you receive an urgent page to come to this patient. Figure 9-18 shows the current flow-volume loop.

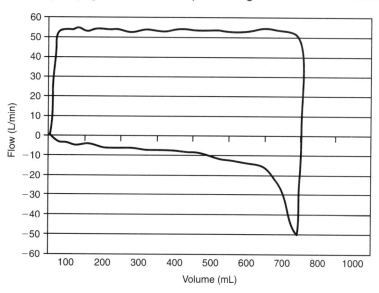

10. Explain the difference between the two flow-volume loops in Figure 9-18.

_____

11. What is the most likely cause of this difference?

_____

12. What therapeutic intervention should you recommend for this patient?

_____

1. In the pressure-time scalar shown in Figure 9-19, line *A* represents which of the following?

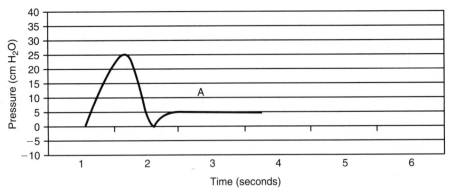

a. Intrinsic PEEP
b. $P_{plateau}$
c. PS
d. Transairway pressure

2. In the pressure-time scalar shown in Figure 9-20, the difference between curve *A* and curve *B* is due to which of the following?

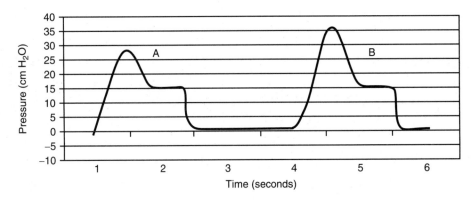

1. Atelectasis
2. Bronchospasm
3. Increased airway secretions
4. Pulmonary edema

a. 1 and 2
b. 1 and 3
c. 2 and 3
d. 2 and 4

3. Using curve *B* in Figure 9-20, calculate the R_{aw} if the set inspiratory flow rate is 40 L/min.
a. 0.5 cm H_2O/L/s
b. 2 cm H_2O/L/s
c. 30 cm H_2O/L/s
d. 52 cm H_2O/L/s

4. The problem with the pressure-time scalar shown in Figure 9-21 is which of the following?

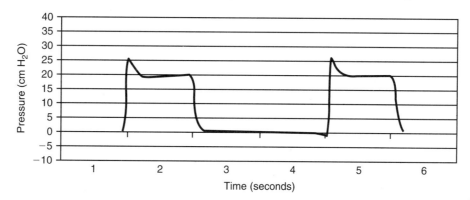

a. Patient is actively exhaling
b. Pressure rise is too rapid
c. Sensitivity setting is incorrect
d. Inspiratory pause is too long

5. Correction of the problem identified in Question 4 includes which of the following?
a. Shorten the T_I
b. Reduce the sensitivity
c. Adjust the inspiratory slope
d. Eliminate the inspiratory pause

6. During PSV for a patient with COPD, the respiratory therapist notices a pressure increase toward the end of inspiration on the pressure-time scalar. This phenomenon can be corrected by which of the following?
a. Shorten the set inspiratory time
b. Increase the flow cycle percent
c. Lower the set PS level
d. Increase the inspiratory flow setting

7. A pressure-volume loop during VC-CMV extends farther to the right and flattens out with which of the following conditions?
a. Pneumonia
b. Bronchitis
c. Asthma
d. Emphysema

8. A flow-volume loop is incomplete because the volume does not return to zero. This can be caused by which of the following conditions?
a. Air trapping
b. Flow starvation
c. Bronchopleural fistula
d. Overdistention of alveoli

Chapter **9 Ventilator Graphics**

9. The pressure-time scalar for VC-CMV shown in Figure 9-22 demonstrates which of the following problems?

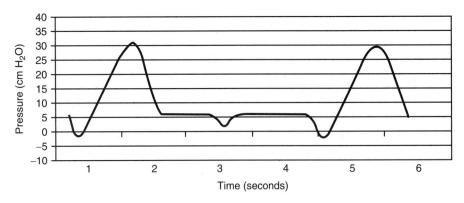

a. Flow starvation
b. Active exhalation
c. Patient-ventilator dyssynchrony
d. Incorrect sensitivity setting

10. The flow-volume loop for VC-CMV shown in Figure 9-23 demonstrates which of the following problems?

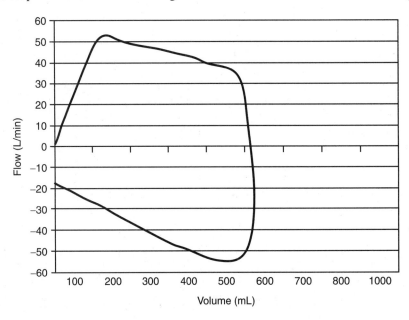

a. Atelectasis
b. Intrinsic PEEP
c. Flow starvation
d. Bronchopleural fistula

HELPFUL INTERNET SITES

- Critical Care Medicine Tutorials, A System for Analyzing Ventilator Waveforms
  http://www.ccmtutorials.com/rs/mv/page15.htm
- Drager Medical
  http://www.draeger.com/media/10/08/41/10084127/rsp_curves_and_loops_booklet_9097421_en.pdf
- C. S. Williams, "Ventilator Graphics ver. 3.0"
  http://www.scribd.com/doc/19584228/Ventilator-Graphics

10 Assessment of Respiratory Function

Upon completion of this chapter, the reader will be able to do the following:

1. Describe the principle of operation of the pulse oximeter.
2. Identify conditions that can influence the accuracy of pulse oximetry readings.
3. Name the test used to determine disparities between arterial oxygen saturation (S_aO_2), arterial oxyhemoglobin saturation (SpO_2), and the patient's clinical condition.
4. Discuss the normal components of a capnogram.
5. Give examples of pathophysiologic conditions that can alter the contour of the capnogram.
6. Identify the normal value for arterial to end-tidal partial pressure of carbon dioxide ($P[a\text{-}et]CO_2$).
7. Describe the various components of a volumetric CO_2 tracing, and discuss how these types of tracings can be used to assess gas exchange during mechanical ventilation.
8. Explain the theory of operation of transcutaneous PO_2 and PCO_2 monitors.
9. List the clinical data that should be recorded when making transcutaneous measurements.
10. Describe the major components of an indirect calorimeter.
11. Provide the respiratory quotient (RQ) value associated with substrate utilization patterns in normal, healthy subjects.
12. Discuss some clinical applications of metabolic monitoring in critically ill patients.
13. Briefly describe devices that are used to measure airway pressures, volumes, and flows during mechanical ventilation.
14. Calculate mean airway pressure, dynamic compliance, static compliance, and airway resistance.
15. Identify pathologic conditions that alter lung compliance and airway resistance.
16. Describe how changes in airway resistance and respiratory system compliance will affect the results of measurements of the work of breathing.
17. Define *pressure-time product*, and discuss its application in the management of mechanically ventilated patients.

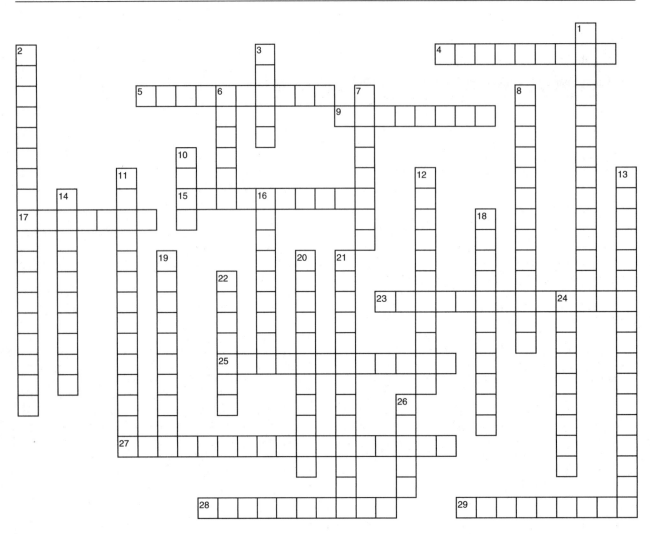

Across

4 The type of pressure measured by occluding the airway during the first 100 ms of a patient's spontaneous inspiration
5 A method of sampling respired gases that extracts gas from the airway through a narrow plastic tube to the measuring chamber, which is located in a separate console
9 The type of dead space free of carbon dioxide
15 Opposition to airflow
17 The type of pressure that reflects alveolar pressure
23 A continuous, noninvasive method of assessing arterial oxygen saturation (two words)
25 Qualitative estimates of exhaled carbon dioxide are made with a _____ detector
27 Relies on the Beer-Lambert Law
28 The type of hemoglobin that is calculated by dividing the oxyhemoglobin concentration by concentration of hemoglobin capable of carrying oxygen
29 A breakdown product of heme metabolism that causes a yellow discoloration of the skin

Down

1 A term used to describe the movement factor that may affect pulse oximetry readings
2 The difference between gastric and esophageal pressures
3 A complication that can occur with the patient's skin when using transcutaneous monitoring
6 A medical condition that can cause an increase in carbon dioxide production
7 An estimation of energy expenditure from measurements of oxygen consumption and carbon dioxide production is known as _____ calorimetry
8 A term used to describe states of low perfusion
10 Force times distance
11 Monitoring at the skin surface is known as _____ monitoring
12 Abnormally low circulating blood volume
13 The type of hemoglobin that has carbon monoxide attached to it

Down—Cont'd

14 A type of device that samples respired gases whose sampling chamber attaches directly to the endotracheal tube and analysis is performed at the airway

16 The shape of the oxyhemoglobin dissociation curve

18 The measurement of carbon dioxide concentration in respired gases

19 Lung volume achieved for a given amount of applied pressure

20 Instrument accuracy depends on this

21 Absorbs more light at 940 nm

22 Cyclical changes in light transmission allows _____ plethysmography to estimate pulse rate

24 _____ CO_2 monitoring focuses on exhaled CO_2 plotted over time, whereas volumetric capnometry focuses on exhaled CO_2 plotted relative to exhaled volume (hyphenated word)

26 The type of hemoglobin that absorbs both red and infrared light (abbreviation)

CHAPTER REVIEW QUESTIONS

1. List five ways to noninvasively monitoring the respiratory function of mechanically ventilated patients.

    a. _____

    b. _____

    c. _____

    d. _____

    e. _____

2. List four causes commonly associated with hypoxemic events in mechanically ventilated patients.

    a. _____

    b. _____

    c. _____

    d. _____

3. Name four sites where a pulse oximetry sensor can be placed.

    a. _____

    b. _____

    c. _____

    d. _____

4. The two principles on which pulse oximetry is based are _____ and _____

5. How is oxyhemoglobin and deoxyhemoglobin differentiated by pulse oximetry?

    _____

    _____

    _____

    _____

6. How is pulse rate determined by a pulse oximeter?

    _____

    _____

    _____

    _____

    _____

7. What determines the accuracy of any diagnostic instrument?

    _____

8. Based on the SpO_2 reading, when should an arterial blood gas (ABG) be drawn to confirm the patient's oxygen saturation?

    _____

9. Identify four conditions that can influence the accuracy of pulse oximetry readings.

    a. _____

    b. _____

    c. _____

    d. _____

10. List three factors that contribute to low perfusion states in patients.

    a. _____

    b. _____

    c. _____

11. The four types of hemoglobin that adult blood typically contains are:

   a. _____

   b. _____

   c. _____

   d. _____

12. Describe the difference between fractional hemoglobin saturation and functional hemoglobin saturation.

   _____

   _____

   _____

   _____

13. When carboxyhemoglobin (COHb) is present in the blood what happens to the SpO_2? _____

14. What medications can cause methemoglobin (MetHb) presence in the blood?

   _____

   _____

15. Describe the effect MetHb has on SpO_2 measurements.

   _____

   _____

16. How can nail polish affect SpO_2? What term is used to describe this possible complication?

   _____

   _____

17. What affect does skin pigmentation have on SpO_2?

   _____

   _____

18. What test is used to determine disparities among SpO_2, SaO_2, and a patient's clinical presentation?

   _____

   _____

   _____

19. The continuous display of carbon dioxide concentrations as a graphic waveform is called a

   _____

20. Describe a specific clinical situation in which chemical capnometer, or colorimetric detector, would be particularly useful.

   _____

   _____

   _____

21. What affect does the presence of water vapor and nitrous oxide have on the accuracy of CO_2 measurements?

   _____

   _____

   _____

22. Describe the two methods of gas sampling used by infrared analyzers.

   a. _____

   b. _____

23. The normal percentage of CO_2 in expired air is.

   _____

24. Identify and explain the labeled parts of Figure 10-1.

   A. _____

   B. _____

   C. _____

   D. _____

   E. _____

25. What determines the amount of CO_2 produced by a patient? Explain.

   _____

   _____

   _____

26. What pathophysiologic conditions can increase or decrease a patient's metabolic rate?

   _____

   _____

   _____

27. For a normal individual, what is the relationship between $PetCO_2$ and P_aCO_2?

   _____

   _____

28. What pathophysiologic conditions cause a decrease in ventilation relative to perfusion, thereby causing a higher than normal $PetCO_2$?

   _____

   _____

29. Where is the lowest $PetCO_2$ reading in the lungs found?

   _____

   _____

30. What pathophysiologic conditions cause a decrease in perfusion relative to ventilation, thereby causing a lower than normal $PetCO_2$?

   _____

   _____

   _____

31. List four pathophysiologic conditions that can alter the contour of a capnogram.

   a. _____

   b. _____

   c. _____

   d. _____

32. What do the labeled capnogram waveforms in Figure 10-2 represent?

   A. _____

   B. _____

   C. _____

33. What pathologic condition can mimic esophageal intubation identified by capnography?

   _____

   _____

34. Describe a situation that may cause gastric PCO_2 to be at almost normal $PetCO_2$ levels.

   _____

   _____

35. Measuring the CO_2 at the end of a forced vital capacity is called the _____.

36. What should the $P(a\text{-}et)CO_2$ measurement be during normal tidal breathing?

   _____

   _____

37. What do the x- and y-axis represent in a volumetric CO_2 tracing?

   _____

   _____

38. Identify and explain the phases represented by the letters in Figure 10-3, which displays a single breath CO_2 curve.

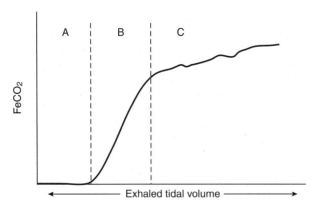

A. _____
_____

B. _____
_____

C. _____
_____

39. Label all the blanks in Figure 10-4.

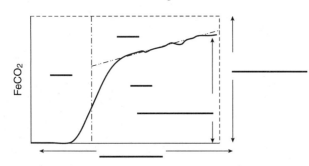

40. Explain the three areas of a volumetric CO_2 tracing.

a. _____

b. _____

c. _____

41. What are the four major events that influence the way CO_2 is exhaled through the lungs?

a. _____

b. _____

c. _____

d. _____

42. How can trending $\dot{V}CO_2$ be used during the weaning process?

_____
_____
_____
_____
_____

43. Why is the monitoring of exhaled NO useful in the management of severe asthma?

_____
_____
_____

44. What type of electrode is used in a transcutaneous oxygen monitor?

_____
_____

45. Why is the transcutaneous oxygen probe heated?

_____
_____
_____
_____

46. Describe a patient population that is best suited for transcutaneous oxygen monitoring.

_____
_____

47. List five causes of erroneous $PtcO_2$ readings.

a. _____

b. _____

c. _____

d. _____

e. _____

48. What type of electrode is used for transcutaneous carbon dioxide measurements?

_____
_____

49. What affect does heating the transcutaneous carbon dioxide probe have on the measurements?

_____

_____

_____

50. How often should the transcutaneous electrode and sensor membrane be changed?

_____

_____

_____

51. What steps should be taken when placing a transcutaneous electrode on the patient's skin?

_____

_____

_____

_____

52. The high and low values for a 2-point calibration of a transcutaneous oxygen monitor are

_____ and _____.

53. The high and low values for a 2-point calibration of a transcutaneous carbon dioxide monitor are

_____ and _____.

54. List the clinical data that should be documented when making transcutaneous measurements.

_____

_____

_____

_____

_____

55. How often should a transcutaneous sensor be repositioned?

_____

56. What device is most commonly used to perform indirect calorimetry?

_____

57. Describe the major components of an indirect calorimeter.

_____

_____

_____

_____

_____

_____

58. What position should the patient be in and for how long before making an indirect calorimetry measurement?

_____

_____

59. The room temperature should be between

_____ and _____ when obtaining indirect calorimetry readings.

60. Why is a urinary nitrogen level necessary for calculating energy expenditure?

_____

_____

_____

61. What is the energy expenditure (EE) of a normal healthy adult?

_____

62. A hypermetabolic state exists when EE is

_____, and a hypometabolic state

exists when EE is _____.

63. List seven [A1]conditions that cause hypermetabolic states and five conditions that cause hypometabolic states.

_____

_____

_____

_____

_____

_____

_____

_____

_____

_____

64. What is the RQ range for a healthy adult consuming a typical American diet?

_____

65. The RQ for feedings of large amounts of glucose is

and for prolonged starvation is _____.

66. When CO_2 production increases, what happens to the respiratory quotient?

_____

67. How can diet influence a patient's failure to wean from mechanical ventilatory support?

_____

_____

_____

_____

68. The devices used to measure airway pressures in the current generation of adult and neonatal ventilators

are _____

69. Which flow-measuring device can be used to detect bidirectional flow?

_____

70. What are some potential caused for increases in peak inspiratory pressure (PIP)?

_____

_____

71. What is the formula for calculating mean airway pressure?

_____

72. Work to overcome the normal elastic and resistive forces plus the work to overcome a disease process affecting normal workloads in the lung and thorax is

known as_____.

73. List five factors that increase the extrinsic work of breathing.

a. _____

b. _____

c. _____

d. _____

e. _____

74. What is the mathematical formula for the work of breathing?

_____

75. Describe how increases in airway resistance will affect the results of measurements of the work of breathing.

_____

_____

_____

76. How can a decrease in static compliance affect the patient's work of breathing?

_____

_____

_____

_____

77. List five pathologic conditions that are associated with decreases in lung compliance.

a. _____

b. _____

c. _____

d. _____

e. _____

78. What condition is associated with reductions in both C_{STAT} and C_{DYN}?

_____

_____

79. What pathologic conditions are associated with increases in airway resistance?

_____

_____

_____

80. What is transdiaphragmatic pressure and how is it measured?

_____

_____

_____

_____

81. What is the pressure-time product?

_____

_____

_____

_____

82. What is occlusion pressure and how is it measured?

_____

_____

_____

CRITICAL THINKING QUESTIONS

1. Why does pulse oximetry become unreliable when dysfunctional hemoglobins (COHb and MetHb) are present in a patient's blood?

_____

_____

_____

_____

_____

2. When trying to use a finger probe for pulse oximetry, the respiratory therapist finds that pulse rate and the electrocardiogram monitor are not consistent and there is no SpO_2 reading. The patient does not have on nail polish. What are the two most likely causes of this problem and what could be done to correct them?

_____

_____

_____

_____

_____

_____

3. What affect does cardiac arrest and decreased cardiac output have on CO_2 detection?

_____

_____

_____

_____

_____

_____

4. Given the following information, determine whether the patient is in a normal, hypermetabolic, or hypometabolic state. The patient is a 48-year-old female, weight 170 pounds, height 5 feet 7 inches, measured CO_2 production is 380 mL/min, and oxygen consumption is 420 mL/min.

_____

_____

_____

_____

_____

_____

_____

_____

_____

_____

_____

Case Study 1

A respiratory therapist is assessing a patient receiving mechanical ventilatory support in the intensive care unit. The pulse oximeter attached to the patient is reading SpO_2 of 74%. The patient's F_IO_2 is set at 0.40.

1. Is the pulse oximeter reading accurate? Why or why not?

_____

_____

2. The patient's physician asks the respiratory therapist for a recommendation as to which laboratory studies to order to clarify or confirm the pulse oximeter reading. What studies are appropriate for this patient at this time?

_____

_____

Case Study 2

A patient is brought to the emergency department following an apartment fire. The patient is brought in receiving oxygen from a nonrebreathing mask. Because there are facial burns, the patient is intubated and placed on mechanical ventilatory support with the F_IO_2 set at 0.50. The pulse oximeter is reading 99%.

1. Is the pulse oximeter reading accurate? Why or why not?

_____

_____

An ABG analysis shows an oxygen saturation of 95% while receiving an F_IO_2 of 0.50.

2. Is this saturation accurate? Why or why not?

_____

_____

3. In this situation, what lab test should be suggested and why?

_____

_____

Case Study 3

A patient is in the process of being weaned from mechanical ventilatory support and is in the SIMV-VC mode and is being monitored with end-tidal CO_2. The respiratory therapist has just decreased the ventilator rate to 4 breaths/min; the set V_T is 500 mL. In Figure 10-5, *A* and *B*, show the tracings that occurred after this change.

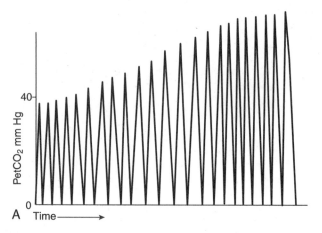

A

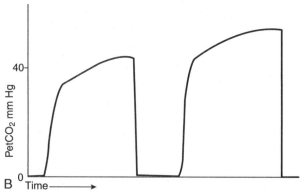

B

1. Analyze both the CO_2 trend and waveform.

_____

_____

2. What are the possible causes for the CO_2 trend?

_____

_____

The respiratory therapist observes the patient using accessory muscles during spontaneous breathing. In addition, there is a decreasing spontaneous tidal volume and increasing spontaneous respiratory rate.

3. How do these findings correlate with the $PetCO_2$ findings?

_____

_____

_____

4. How can the problem be alleviated?

_____

_____

Case Study 4

A respiratory therapist is monitoring the arterial to maximum end-expiratory PCO_2 difference for a patient with chronic obstructive pulmonary disease (COPD) who is receiving mechanical ventilatory support. Over the past 24 hours, the $P(a\text{-}et)CO_2$ has increased from 5 to 18 mm Hg.

1. Is this increase one that is expected for a patient with COPD? Why or why not?

_____

_____

2. What would a single breath CO_2 curve look like for this situation?

_____

_____

_____

NBRC-STYLE QUESTIONS

1. A pulse oximeter is generally considered accurate for oxygen saturations greater than which of the following?
   a. 65%
   b. 70%
   c. 75%
   d. 80%

2. A respiratory therapist encounters a patient whose pulse oximetry reading is 73%. The most appropriate action is which of the following?
   a. Change the sensor and move it to a different location.
   b. Contact the patient's physician for further instructions.
   c. Confirm the value with arterial blood CO-oximeter analysis.
   d. Accept the value and record it in the patient's medical record.

3. Which of the following most directly affects the response time of a pulse oximeter?
   a. The type of pulse oximeter
   b. The location of the sensor or probe
   c. The percentage of oxygen saturation
   d. The position of the patient in the bed

4. The oxyhemoglobin concentration divided by the concentration of hemoglobin capable of carrying oxygen determines which of the following?
   a. Dysfunctional hemoglobin
   b. Fractional hemoglobin
   c. Functional hemoglobin
   d. Methemoglobin

5. On rounds, a respiratory therapist encounters a patient who is receiving supplemental oxygen and whose SpO_2 is constantly displaying 85%. The respiratory therapist notes that the patient is also receiving dapsone. Which of the following is the most appropriate action to take?
   a. Use an ear lobe probe for more accuracy.
   b. Contact the patient's physician for further instructions.
   c. Confirm the value with arterial blood CO-oximeter analysis.
   d. Accept the value and record it in the patient's medical record.

6. The partial pressure of end-tidal carbon dioxide is read at what point on a capnogram?
   a. During phase 1
   b. End of phase 2
   c. During phase 3
   d. End of phase 4

7. The arterial to *maximum* expiratory PCO_2 gradient will be greatest for a patient with which of the following?
   a. COPD
   b. Asthma
   c. Left-sided heart failure
   d. Pulmonary embolism

8. The most reliable method for ruling out esophageal intubation is which of the following?
   a. Presence of CO_2 in the patient's exhaled gas
   b. Presence of condensation in the endotracheal tube
   c. Presence of bilateral breath sounds on auscultation
   d. Increased resistance to squeezing the manual resuscitator bag

9. Most likely, cardiac arrest will cause a colorimetric CO_2 detector to display which of the following?
   a. Less than 1% CO_2
   b. 1%-2% CO_2
   c. 2%-5% CO_2
   d. Greater than 5% CO_2

10. A respiratory therapist is called to the bedside of a patient who is being transcutaneously monitored for PO_2 and PCO_2. The signal is drifting and will not stabilize during calibration. The most appropriate action includes which of the following?
    1. Recalibrate the monitor with 15 and 20% CO_2.
    2. Clean the electrode and change the sensor membrane.
    3. Remove excess electrolyte solution from the electrode surface.
    4. Add a drop of electrolyte solution to the electrode surface.
    a. 1 and 2 only
    b. 1 and 3 only
    c. 2 and 4 only
    d. 3 and 4 only

11. A difficult to wean patient with COPD has an RQ of 0.98. The most likely cause of this patient's inability to be weaned is which of the following?
    a. Reliance on lipid metabolism is causing hypoxemia.
    b. Lipogenesis is causing the patient to retain CO_2.
    c. A highly restricted carbohydrate metabolism is generating hypoxia.
    d. Excessive carbohydrates are overloading the patient's ventilatory reserve.

12. The tracing of a slow-speed capnograph is not returning to zero every exhalation. The most likely cause of this finding is which of the following?
    a. The F_IO_2 was decreased.
    b. The patient is hyperventilating.
    c. CO_2 is being rebreathed.
    d. The capnograph needs to be recalibrated.

13. A respiratory therapist monitoring a patient receiving mechanical ventilatory support finds that over the past 2 hours the patient's PIP is increasing but the static pressure has remained stable. Which of the following could cause this?
    a. Atelectasis
    b. Pneumothorax
    c. Retained secretions
    d. Right mainstem intubation

14. Which of the following will increase intrinsic work of breathing?
    a. Bronchospasm
    b. Endotracheal tube
    c. Machine sensitivity
    d. Heat moisture exchanger

15. Figure 10-6 is indicative of which of the following?

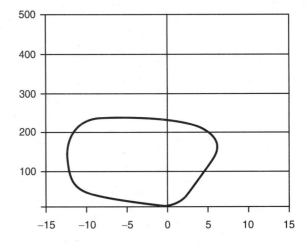

    a. Mechanical breath with little work of breathing
    b. Spontaneous breath under normal circumstances
    c. Spontaneous breath with high impedance to breathing
    d. Patient breathing through a freestanding continuous positive airway pressure system

11 Hemodynamic Monitoring

LEARNING OBJECTIVES

Upon completion of this chapter, the reader will be able to do the following:

1. Discuss how changes in heart rate (HR), preload, contractility, and afterload can alter cardiac function and cardiac output.
2. Identify indicators of left ventricular preload, contractility, and afterload.
3. Name the major components of a hemodynamic monitoring system.
4. Explain the proper technique for the insertion and maintenance of a systemic arterial line, and list the most common complications that can occur with this type of monitoring system.
5. Describe the procedures for the insertion and placement of a central venous line, a balloon flotation, and a flow-directed pulmonary artery catheter, and list the potential complications associated with these devices.
6. Interpret the waveforms generated during the insertion of a pulmonary artery catheter.
7. Calculate arterial and venous oxygen content, cardiac output, cardiac index, stroke index, cardiac cycle time, left ventricular stroke work index (LVSWI), right ventricular stroke work index (RVSWI), and pulmonary and systemic vascular resistance.
8. List normal values for measured and derived hemodynamic variables.
9. Describe the most common complications associated with pulmonary artery catheterization and discuss strategies that can be used to minimize these complications.
10. Compare the effects of spontaneous and mechanical ventilation breathing on hemodynamic values.
11. Define the following terms: *incisura*, *pulse pressure*, *stroke index*, *stroke work*, *systemic vascular resistance (SVR)*, *pulmonary vascular resistance (PVR)*, and *ejection fraction*.
12. Explain how measurements of pulmonary capillary wedge pressure can be used to evaluate left ventricular function.
13. Differentiate between cardiogenic and noncardiogenic pulmonary edema using hemodynamic parameters.
14. From a patient case, describe how hemodynamic monitoring can be used in the diagnosis and treatment of selected cases of critically ill patients.

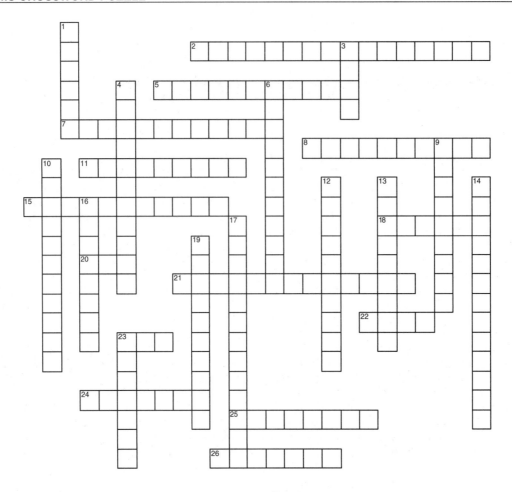

Across

2 Ratio of the stroke volume to the ventricular end-diastolic volume (two words)
5 Type of pressure exerted by a fluid while it is at a standstill
7 Type of pressure exerted by a fluid while it is in motion
8 Fluid flowing in the opposite direction
11 One of the atrioventricular valves
15 Heart rates less than 60 beats/min
18 Valve between the left atrium and left ventricle
20 The afterload that the left ventricle must overcome to eject blood into the systemic circulation (abbreviation)
21 Type of catheter line that is inserted into the right atrium (two words)
22 Another name for pulmonary capillary wedge pressure (abbreviation)
23 The afterload that the right ventricle must overcome to eject blood into the pulmonary circulation (abbreviation)
24 A pulmonary artery catheter floats because of this
25 Small negative deflection on the aortic and pulmonary artery tracing
26 Contraction that causes ejection of blood from the heart

Down

1 The unit for pulmonary artery catheter size
3 Principle used to calculate cardiac output
4 Quantification of the amount of pressure generated by the heart during systole (two words)
6 HRs greater than 100 beats/min
9 Impedance that the left and right ventricles must overcome to eject blood into the great vessels
10 Stroke volume divided by body surface area (two words)
12 Work done by the ventricle to eject a volume of blood into the aorta (two words)
13 Both the aortic and pulmonary valves are this type of valve
14 Difference between the systolic and diastolic pressures (two words)
16 Cardiac relaxation and filling
17 Pumping strength of the heart
19 A type of electrical bridge used in pressure transducers
23 Filling pressure of the ventricle at the end of ventricular diastole

CHAPTER REVIEW QUESTIONS

1. List four common invasive hemodynamic measurements.

   a. _____

   b. _____

   c. _____

   d. _____

2. What is the primary indication for hemodynamic monitoring?

   _____

3. When the heart rate is 90 beats/min, what is the length of one cardiac cycle?

   _____

4. What typically causes retrograde flow in the heart?

   _____

5. Define *afterload*.

   _____

   _____

6. What resistance must the left ventricle overcome to pump blood systemically?

   _____

7. What resistance must the right ventricle overcome to pump blood to the lungs?

   _____

   _____

   _____

8. During atrial systole, which heart valves are open and which are closed?

   _____

   _____

9. What is the term used to describe pressure exerted while a fluid is (a) in motion and (b) not in motion?

   a. _____

   b. _____

10. Where should a transducer be placed to measure accurately?

    _____

11. What happens to the pressure measurement if the transducer is (a) higher than the catheter tip and (b) lower than the catheter tip?

    a. _____

    b. _____

12. What four main factors influence the outputs of the right and left ventricle?

    a. _____

    b. _____

    c. _____

    d. _____

13. Define *preload*.

    _____

    _____

14. Describe how ventricular systole occurs.

    _____

    _____

    _____

    _____

    _____

    _____

15. What measurements are used to estimate right ventricular end-diastolic pressure and left ventricular end-diastolic pressure?

    _____

    _____

16. What do systemic vascular and pulmonary vascular resistances reflect?

    _____

    _____

17. List the major components of a hemodynamic monitoring system.

_____

_____

_____

_____

18. The mid-thoracic line of the patient is called the

_____ and is used to perform

a _____ on the transducer.

19. Why is positioning of the transducer important for accurate measurements?

_____

_____

_____

_____

20. Explain the proper technique for the insertion and maintenance of a systemic radial arterial line.

_____

_____

_____

_____

_____

_____

21. What are the potential complications that can occur following placement of an arterial catheter line?

_____

_____

22. What type of fluid is used to flush an arterial line? How fast should the flow be set?

_____

_____

23. What factors increase the risk of infection with an arterial line?

_____

_____

24. What potential problem can occur with prolonged or frequent flushing of an arterial line in a neonate or pediatric patient weighing less than 20 kg?

_____

25. List the uses of a central venous line.

_____

_____

26. When a central venous pressure (CVP) measurement is taken at the end of ventricular diastole, what pressure is being estimated?

_____

_____

27. The veins typically used for the insertion of a CVP

line are _____.

28. CVP measurements are usually taken during which phase of breathing and in what position?

_____

29. Common problems and potential complications from central venous line insertion include a:

_____

_____.

30. The normal value range for CVP is _____.

31. What are the pediatric and adult pulmonary artery catheter lengths and available sizes? How are they marked off for insertion purposes?

_____

_____

32. How are clots avoided in a pulmonary artery catheter?

_____

_____

33. Identify the structures, lettered *A* through *G* in Figure 11-1, on a four-channel pulmonary artery catheter.

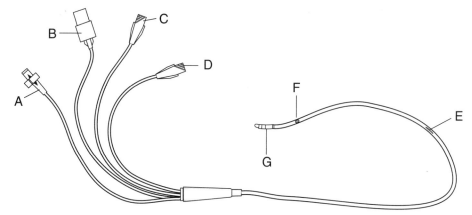

A. _____

B. _____

C. _____

D. _____

E. _____

F. _____

G. _____

34. List the insertion sites, both percutaneous and surgical cut-down, for the insertion of a pulmonary artery catheter.

_____

_____

35. List eight complications associated with pulmonary artery catheterization. Include the cause of each complication.

a. _____

b. _____

c. _____

d. _____

e. _____

f. _____

g. _____

h. _____

36. What are the two ways to determine catheter position during insertion?

a. _____

b. _____

37. Trace the insertion of a pulmonary artery catheter from an internal jugular vein to a pulmonary vein. When is the balloon inflated? Into which lung zone should the catheter be placed?

_____

_____

_____

38. Why does the pulmonary artery catheter need to be placed in the particular zone described in Question 37?

_____

_____

_____

_____

39. What are the pressure relationships in each lung zone?

Zone	Pressure Relationship
1	_____
2	_____
3	_____

40. The volume of an adult pulmonary artery catheter balloon is _____ and should be inflated for only _____ seconds when measuring pulmonary artery occlusion pressure (PAOP).

41. Identify the position of the catheter represented by the letters *A* through *D* in Figure 11-2.

Time (seconds)

A. _____

B. _____

C. _____

D. _____

42. How can you minimize the following problems associated with pulmonary artery catheterization?

a. Ventricular arrhythmias _____

b. Pulmonary artery infarction _____

_____

c. Pulmonary artery rupture _____

d. Balloon rupture _____

43. Explain the relationship between heart rates above 200 beats/min and a decrease in cardiac output.

_____

44. What happens to systemic arterial diastolic pressure when vasoconstriction occurs?

_____

45. Arterial systolic and diastolic pressures are affected by _____ and _____.

46. During what part of the breathing cycle should pulmonary artery pressure be measured?

_____

47. What effect does positive end-expiratory pressure (PEEP) or auto-PEEP at levels above 15 cm H_2O have on PAOP?

_____

48. List three pathologic conditions that increase PVR and subsequently pulmonary artery pressure (PAP).

a. _____

b. _____

c. _____

49. What effect does inhaled nitric oxide have on the pulmonary vasculature?

_____

_____

50. Compare the effects of spontaneous breathing to mechanical ventilation as it relates to pulmonary artery pressure.

_____

_____

51. Complete the table below with the appropriate hemodynamic values.

Parameter	Normal Value
Arterial blood pressure	_____
Mean arterial pressure	_____
Pulse pressure	_____
CVP	_____
PAP	_____
Pulmonary artery wedge pressure (PAWP)	_____

52. Complete the following chart with the formulas used to calculate each value.

Calculate Value	Formula	Normal Values
Cardiac output	_____	_____
Cardiac index	_____	_____
Stroke index	_____	_____
Arterial oxygen content	_____	_____
Mixed venous oxygen content	_____	_____
SVR	_____	_____
PVR	_____	_____

53. What are the effects of the following factors on cardiac output?

Factor	Effect on Cardiac Output
Tachycardia	_____
Beta-adrenergic blockade	_____
Increased parasympathetic tone	_____
Increased preload and contractility	_____
Bradycardia	_____
Decreased parasympathetic tone	_____

For Questions 54 through 57, calculate oxygen content given the information in each question.

54. P_aO_2 43 mm Hg, S_aO_2 75%, hemoglobin (Hb) 10 g%

_____

_____

55. P_aO_2 64 mm Hg, S_aO_2 94%, Hb 13 g%

_____

_____

56. P_vO_2 40 mm Hg, S_vO_2 75%, Hb 15 g%

_____

_____

57. P_vO_2 70 mm Hg, S_vO_2 85%, Hb 16 g%

_____

_____

58. Explain why mixed venous oxygen values decrease when cardiac output is reduced.

_____

_____

59. What are the two most important factors that influence vascular resistance? Give examples of each.

a. _____

b. _____

60. What effect does alveolar hypoxia and high intra-alveolar pressures have on PVR?

_____

61. List three mathematically derived indicators of left ventricular contractility.

a. _____

b. _____

c. _____

CRITICAL THINKING QUESTIONS

1. Explain how measurements of pulmonary capillary occlusion pressure can be used to evaluate left ventricular function.

   _____

   _____

   _____

   _____

   _____

   _____

2. Differentiate between cardiogenic and noncardiogenic pulmonary edema using hemodynamic parameters.

   _____

   _____

   _____

   _____

   _____

   _____

   _____

   _____

   _____

3. Define pulse pressure. What conditions can lead to (a) an increased pulse pressure and (b) a decreased pulse pressure?

   a. _____

   _____

   b. _____

   _____

   _____

111

Case Study 1

A 53-year-old, 6-foot tall, 195-lb male was admitted for head trauma due to a motor vehicle accident. In the operating room, the patient had a craniotomy to relieve pressure. He is currently in the surgical intensive care unit receiving mechanical ventilation with VC-SIMV, rate 8, V_T 650 mL, and F_IO_2 0.6. The patient is receiving dobutamine. A pulmonary artery catheter is inserted and the following information is collected:

PAP: 38/20 mm Hg   CVP: 12 mm Hg   HR: 92 b/min
PAWP: 10 mm Hg   BP: 145/68 mm Hg   Hb: 12.6 g%
CO: 5.1 L/min

	Arterial Blood Gas	Mixed Venous Gas
pH	7.46	7.38
PCO_2	32 mm Hg	43 mm Hg
P_aO_2	100 mm Hg	40 mm Hg
S_aO_2	99%	75%

Calculate the following and indicate whether normal, high, or low:

1. Pulse pressure _____

2. Stroke volume _____

3. Stroke index _____

4. Cardiac index _____

5. Mean arterial pressure _____

6. Mean pulmonary artery pressure _____

7. SVR _____

8. PVR _____

9. C_aO_2 _____

10. C_vO_2 _____

11. C(a-v)O_2 _____

12. DO_2 _____

13. VO_2 _____

14. RVSW _____

15. RVSWI _____

16. LVSW _____

17. LVSWI _____

18. Comment on the patient data.

_____

_____

_____

Case Study 2

The respiratory therapist is monitoring a patient who is receiving mechanical ventilatory support in one of the intensive care units. Hemodynamic monitoring of this patient is being considered because of patient instability.

1. What aspect of hemodynamic monitoring should the respiratory therapist suggest for this patient?

_____

_____

A hemodynamic monitoring system is now in place. The catheter was inserted through the subclavian 1 hour ago. The patient is now exhibiting signs of respiratory distress. Breath sounds are absent on the patient's right side.

2. What complication is most likely causing this clinical situation?

_____

3. What is the most likely cause of this complication?

_____

Following correction of the problem, the PAOP was 12 mm Hg. As the day progressed, however, the pressure rose to 15 mm Hg, and then over the next few hours to 19 mm Hg. The pressure has now stabilized at 25 mm Hg.

4. What is the significance of this finding?

_____

NBRC-STYLE QUESTIONS

1. The respiratory therapist is assisting a physician inserting a pulmonary artery catheter in a patient when it is noted that a dampened or continuous low-pressure waveform is displayed on the oscilloscope. This indicates which of the following?
   a. The catheter is not wedged.
   b. The balloon is deflated and the catheter is not wedged.
   c. The balloon may still be inflated or the catheter may be wedged.
   d. The balloon is deflated and the catheter has perforated the right ventricle.

2. The PAOP value most indicative of cardiogenic pulmonary edema is which of the following?
   a. 8 mm Hg
   b. 12 mm Hg
   c. 18 mm Hg
   d. 25 mm Hg

3. The pressure measured from the proximal lumen of a pulmonary artery catheter is referred to as:
   a. PAP
   b. RAP
   c. RVP
   d. PAWP

4. Which of the following procedures verifies the position of a pulmonary catheter?
   a. Checking the pressure waveform
   b. Checking the number of centimeters inserted
   c. Obtaining a blood sample through the catheter tip
   d. Obtaining a chest radiograph for catheter tip placement

5. The third lumen of a pulmonary artery catheter is used to measure which of the following?
   a. CO
   b. CVP
   c. PAP
   d. PAOP

6. A low CVP value is indicative of which of the following?
   a. Shock, dehydration, or hemorrhage
   b. Shock, overhydration, or hemorrhage
   c. Hypertension, dehydration, or hypervolemia
   d. Hypertension, overhydration, and hypovolemia

7. Which of the following complications is most common following long-term placements of systemic arterial catheterization?
   a. Hemorrhage and spasm of the artery
   b. Cardiac valve stenosis and prolapse
   c. Arterial laceration and subsequent hemorrhage
   d. Infection and tissue ischemia distal to the catheter

8. The proper location for the distal tip of a central venous catheter is in which of the following?
   a. Left ventricle or aorta
   b. Vena cava or right atrium
   c. Right ventricle or pulmonary artery
   d. Pulmonary artery or pulmonary capillary

9. Which of the following measurements may best estimate left ventricular preload?
   a. RAP
   b. CVP
   c. PAP
   d. PAOP

10. Which of the following will increase cardiac index?
    a. Shock
    b. Exercise
    c. Hypovolemia
    d. Cardiac failure

12 Methods to Improve Ventilation in Patient-Ventilator Management

LEARNING OBJECTIVES

Upon completion of this chapter, the reader will be able to do the following:

1. Recommend ventilator adjustments to reduce work of breathing and improve ventilation based on patient diagnosis, arterial blood gas (ABG) results, and ventilator parameters.
2. Calculate the appropriate suction catheter size, length, and amount of suction pressure needed for a specific size endotracheal tube (ET) and patient.
3. Compare the benefits of closed-suction catheters to the open suction technique.
4. List the pros and cons of instilling normal saline to loosen secretions before suctioning.
5. List the clinical findings that are used to establish the presence of a respiratory infection.
6. Compare the protocols for using metered-dose inhalers (MDIs) and small volume nebulizers (SVNs) during mechanical ventilation.
7. Describe complications associated with using SVNs powered by external flowmeters during mechanical ventilation.
8. Discuss the importance of patient-centered mechanical ventilation in the treatment of critically ill patients.
9. Discuss the complications associated with the in-house transport of a mechanically ventilated patient.

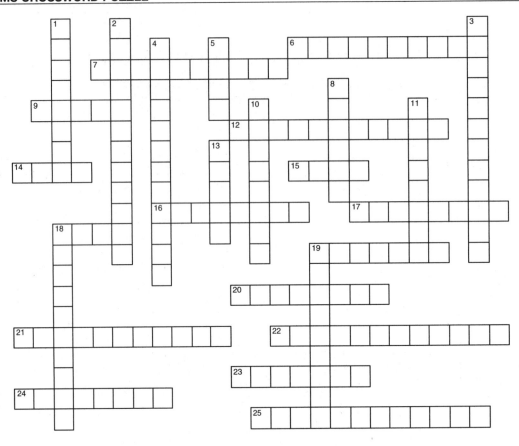

Across

6 _____ overdose can cause metabolic acidosis
7 Caused by a medical procedure or treatment
9 Fever, multiple trauma, sepsis, and _____ can increase metabolism and CO_2 production
12 Normal ventilation
14 Medication given to keep pH greater than 7.25 (abbreviation)
15 Type of suctioning that can decrease ventilator-associated pneumonias (VAPs) in intubated patients (abbreviation)
16 CO_2 causes vasodilation here
17 Deficient blood flow to the cells
18 Type of aerosol device that delivers puffs of medication (abbreviation)
19 A bag for collecting a patient's exhaled air
20 Rigid tonsil suction tip
21 In pressure-controlled ventilation (PCV) increasing this time will increase volume delivered without increasing pressure
22 "Out of step" with the ventilator
23 A fluid filled with cellular debris and protein that accumulates as a result of inflammation
24 Respiratory acidosis indicates that this type of ventilation is not adequate
25 Part of the standard therapy to reduce intracranial pressure

Down

1 Reduced urinary output
2 Defined as across the pyloric region of the stomach, this type of enteral feeding route reduces the risks of vomiting and aspiration
3 Overhydration causes this effect, which can lead to reduced hemoglobin, hematocrit, and cell counts
4 Procedure for visualizing the bronchi
5 A type of acidosis caused by diabetes, alcoholism, or starvation
8 Suctioning can cause ulceration of the

_____
10 Excessive urinary output
11 Loss of bicarbonate can be caused by

_____
13 A thyroid that is overactive is _____
18 Hypercapnia used to help prevent lung injury
19 Ventilation without perfusion (two words)

Chapter **12 Methods to Improve Ventilation in Patient-Ventilator Management**

CHAPTER REVIEW QUESTIONS

1. Calculate the desired V_T when the known P_aCO_2 is 55 mm Hg, the known V_T is 500 mL, the known frequency is 14, and the desired P_aCO_2 is 40 mm Hg.

2. Calculate the desired frequency when the known P_aCO_2 is 65 mm Hg, the known V_T is 600 mL, the known frequency is 12, and the desired P_aCO_2 is 50 mm Hg.

3. What three factors can affect P_aCO_2 in patients receiving mechanical ventilation?

   a.
   b.
   c.

4. List the three components of an ABG that reflect a patient's ventilatory status.

   a.
   b.
   c.

5. What happens to the $PaCO_2$ and the pH when alveolar ventilation decreases?

6. List six pathologic processes that are associated with acute respiratory acidosis.

   a.
   b.
   c.
   d.
   e.
   f.

7. Explain how volume and pressure affect P_aCO_2 and pH?

8. The recommended target V_T is _____.

9. When increasing V_T it is important to maintain $P_{plateau}$ less than _____.

10. List two methods of increasing V_T in pressure-control ventilation.

    a.
    b.

11. What P_aCO_2 and pH levels typically characterize respiratory alkalosis? _____

12. List seven common causes of respiratory alkalosis.

    a.
    b.
    c.
    d.
    e.
    f.
    g.

13. A patient with a P_aCO_2 of 25 mm Hg and a pH of 7.55 is sedated and ventilated in a volume-controlled mode. Ideal body weight (IBW) is 60 kg. The frequency is set at 18, and the delivered V_T is set at 8 mL/kg. What frequency would result in a P_aCO_2 of 40 mm Hg?

14. Explain how you would correct respiratory alkalosis in a patient during:

    a. Volume-controlled ventilation: _____
    b. PCV: _____

15. A patient on VC-CMV has the frequency set at 10, with the total respiratory rate of 20 breaths/min. The P_aCO_2 is 25 mm Hg with a pH of 7.52. Will decreasing the set rate correct the respiratory alkalosis? Explain your answer.

16. Referring to Question 15, what modes of ventilation may be more appropriate for this patient? Why?

_____

_____

17. List six common causes of hyperventilation in patients receiving mechanical ventilation.

    a. _____

    b. _____

    c. _____

    d. _____

    e. _____

    f. _____

18. What is the body's physiologic response to a metabolic acidosis?

_____

_____

19. List six causes of metabolic acidosis. Give an example of each.

    a. _____

    b. _____

    c. _____

    d. _____

    e. _____

    f. _____

20. What are the pH and bicarbonate levels that typically characterize metabolic acidosis?

_____

21. List five common causes of metabolic alkalosis.

    a. _____

    b. _____

    c. _____

    d. _____

    e. _____

22. What two formulas are used to predict the change in pressure necessary to achieve a desired P_aCO_2?

    a. _____

    b. _____

23. How can mechanical ventilation cause an increase in a patient's dead space?

_____

_____

_____

24. List two examples of pathologic processes that would result in an increase in physiologic dead space.

    a. _____

    b. _____

25. What is the normal range for the V_D/V_T ratio?

_____

_____

26. Calculate the V_D/V_T ratio based on the following information: $V_T = 800$ mL, $P_aCO_2 = 45$ mm Hg, $P_ECO_2 = 36$ mm Hg.

_____

_____

27. List eight clinical disorders that may result in a hypermetabolic state.

    a. _____

    b. _____

    c. _____

    d. _____

    e. _____

    f. _____

    g. _____

    h. _____

28. What effect does hyperventilation have on cerebral blood flow?

_____

29. Describe permissive hypercapnia.

_____

_____

30. What is the effect of permissive hypercapnia on patients with head trauma?

_____

_____

31. List the suction pressure ranges for adults, children, and infants.

_____

_____

32. The maximum length of suction time for an adult is _____ seconds.

33. What is the estimated suction catheter size for a 7.0 ET?

_____

_____

34. List five indications for the endotracheal suctioning of mechanically ventilated patients with artificial airways according to the American Association or Respiratory Care Clinical Practice Guidelines.

a. _____

b. _____

c. _____

d. _____

e. _____

35. Are there any contraindications to suctioning?

_____

36. List nine indications for the use of closed in-line suctioning.

a. _____

b. _____

c. _____

d. _____

e. _____

f. _____

g. _____

h. _____

i. _____

37. Match the complication with its most likely cause.

Complication	Cause
_____ Hypoxemia/hypoxia	a. Suction pressures
_____ Tracheal/mucosal trauma	b. Reduction in lung volume
_____ Cardiac/respiratory arrest	c. Airway trauma
_____ Cardiac arrhythmias	d. Patient or caregiver
_____ Atelectasis	e. Hypoxemia/vagal stimulation
_____ Bronchospasm	f. Extreme response to suctioning and vent disconnect
_____ Infection	g. Ventilator disconnect and loss of positive end-expiratory pressure (PEEP)
_____ Bleeding	h. Reaction to tracheal stimulation

38. Describe presuctioning and postsuctioning procedures as it relates to F_IO_2?

_____

39. List four advantages of closed in-line suction catheter use.

a. _____

b. _____

c. _____

d. _____

40. List five disadvantages of in-line suction catheter use.

a. _____

b. _____

c. _____

d. _____

e. _____

41. List four reasons why silent aspiration and VAP can occur with cuffed ET tubes.

a. _____

b. _____

c. _____

d. _____

42. Describe how silent aspiration and VAP may occur.

_____

_____

_____

43. What is the benefit of using a Hi-Lo Evac ET tube?

_____

_____

_____

44. What pressure should be used with a CASS ET tube?

_____

45. Should you instill saline down the ET before performing endotracheal suctioning? Why or why not?

_____

_____

46. How can ET suctioning be assessed in a patient receiving mechanical ventilation?

_____

_____

_____

47. What parameters should be monitored prior to, during, and after suctioning?

_____

_____

48. Following suctioning of an intubated patient, the respiratory therapist notices that the sputum is rust colored. What is the patient's potential problem?

_____

49. List four patient-related factors influence aerosol deposition in a mechanically ventilated patient.

a. _____

b. _____

c. _____

d. _____

50. List the four types of aerosol-generating devices that can be used to administer aerosolized medications during mechanical ventilation?

a. _____

b. _____

c. _____

d. _____

51. Which mode of mechanical ventilation is thought to be more effective for aerosol delivery?

_____

52. Explain how ventilator tidal volume and respiratory rate affect aerosol delivery.

_____

_____

53. What technical problems with the ventilator are associated with the continuous nebulization using an external gas source?

_____

_____

_____

54. Where in the ventilator circuit should the nebulizers be placed?

_____

_____

55. What three factors would optimize the aerosol deposition of bronchodilators during noninvasive positive-pressure ventilation?

a. _____

b. _____

c. _____

56. List four positive patient responses to bronchodilator therapy during mechanical ventilation.

a. _____

b. _____

c. _____

d. _____

57. A mechanically ventilated patient is given albuterol via pMDI. The pretreatment and post-treatment findings are
Pretreatment: peak inspiratory pressure (PIP) = 32 cm H_2O, $P_{plateau}$ = 8 cm H_2O
Post-treatment: PIP = 23 cm H_2O, $P_{plateau}$ = 10 cm H_2O
Was this treatment effective? Why or why not?

_____

58. What is the goal when performing chest physiotherapy?

_____

_____

59. Chest physiotherapy includes what two procedures?

_____

60. List the sequence of four recommended positions that aid in secretion clearance for ventilated patients.

a. _____

b. _____

c. _____

d. _____

61. List the possible hazards of performing chest physiotherapy on patients requiring mechanical ventilation:

_____

_____

62. List the three channels found in a flexible fiberoptic bronchoscope and the purpose for each.

a. _____

b. _____

c. _____

63. What medication can be given to a ventilated patient prior to a bronchoscopy to reduce secretion production and block the vagal response?

_____

64. What type of patient problem should be suspected when the patient's cardiac output and renal output are decreased and the pulmonary artery occlusions pressure is increased?

_____

65. What is considered normal urinary output?

_____

66. What effect can positive-pressure ventilation have on urinary output?

_____

67. What effect does fluid balance have on blood cell counts?

_____

_____

_____

68. Describe the objective of patient-centered mechanical ventilation.

_____

_____

69. Which ventilator parameters can be adjusted by the respiratory therapist to improve patient comfort?

_____

_____

_____

_____

70. What equipment is needed for the in-house transport of a mechanically ventilated patient?

_____

_____

71. What capabilities should a transport ventilator have to ensure patient safety?

_____

_____

72. List four contraindications to the in-house transport of a mechanically ventilated patient.

a. _____

b. _____

c. _____

d. _____

CRITICAL THINKING QUESTIONS

1. A patient is being ventilated in a volume-controlled mode. The set V_T is 700 mL with a frequency of 10. $P_{plateau}$ equals 45 cm H_2O, and the P_aCO_2 equals 60 mm Hg. The physician would like to reduce the P_aCO_2 to 40 mm Hg but does not want to increase the V_T because of the high $P_{plateau}$. What can the therapist do to decrease the level of P_aCO_2 to 40 mm Hg?

2. A postsurgical patient that suffered trauma following multiple surgical procedures is septic with a fever of 104°F. The patient is being maintained in a volume-controlled mode of ventilation. The V_T is 800 mL, with a set frequency of 15, and the patient is triggering to 25 breaths/min. An ABG reveals a P_aCO_2 of 38 mm Hg, and a P_aO_2 of 42 mm Hg. Why does the patient have a normal P_aCO_2 with a minute ventilation of 20 L/min?

3. A patient in respiratory distress was intubated and placed on pressure-control ventilation with a PEEP level of +5 cm H_2O. Soon after, the patient's cardiac output decreases from 6 to 4.5 L/min. What can the therapist do to help determine what was responsible for the decrease in cardiac output?

CASE STUDIES

Case Study 1

A patient is being ventilated with VC-CMV, rate is 12 breaths/min, V_T is 700 mL, F_IO_2 is 0.5, and PEEP is 5 cm H_2O. The total rate is 25 breaths/min. The pH is 7.52, P_aCO_2 is 30 mm Hg, and P_aO_2 is 45 mm Hg. When the set frequency was reduced to 10 in an attempt to correct the respiratory alkalosis, the total rate remained at 25. An attempt at decreasing the V_T resulted in an increase in the total rate.

1. What can the therapist do to address the respiratory alkalosis for this patient?

Case Study 2

A 100-kg (IBW) patient is receiving PCV with a set pressure of 20 cm H_2O at a frequency of 12 breaths/min. The flow rate reaches zero before the beginning of exhalation. The exhaled volume is 550 mL, P_aCO_2 is 65 mm Hg, and pH is 7.29. The physician requests that the patient's P_aCO_2 be decreased to 45 mm Hg.

1. What would be the most effective means of reducing the patient's P_aCO_2?

2. What parameter change would result in the desired P_aCO_2 of 45 mm Hg?

Case Study 3

A patient with poor compliance is being ventilated in a pressure-controlled mode. The PEEP level is set at 10 cm H_2O with an F_IO_2 of 60. The patient is manually ventilated with 100% O_2 before suctioning. When the ventilator is disconnected from the ET tube and the therapist begins the procedure, there is a rapid drop in O_2 saturation and a marked increase in the heart rate.

1. What is the possible cause of the problem?

2. What can the therapist do to alleviate the situation?

_____

_____

NBRC-STYLE QUESTIONS

1. Which of the following aerosol delivery devices will affect ventilator function when used?
   a. pMDI
   b. USN
   c. SVN
   d. VMN

2. Permissive hypercapnia may be beneficial for a patient with which of the following?
   a. High $P_{plateau}$
   b. Intracranial lesion
   c. Pulmonary hypertension
   d. Head trauma

3. A patient requiring mechanical ventilation has an 8-mm ET in place. The patient requires frequent suctioning and a 10-French catheter is being used. The respiratory therapist should recommend which of the following?
   a. Instill saline with every suctioning procedure
   b. A suction frequency of every 2 hours
   c. Increase the suction pressure to -180 mm Hg
   d. Changing to a size 12-French catheter

4. Which of the following statements pertaining to the Hi-Lo Evac ET is true?
   a. The tube has a suction port at the level of the ET cuff.
   b. The continuous suction pressure should be set at -30 cm H_2O.
   c. The device can reduce the incidence of nosocomial pneumonias.
   d. All patients should have this type of ET tube in place.

5. An 85-kg male (IBW) patient is being ventilated with VC-CMV, $f = 12$ breaths/min, $V_T = 450$ mL. The patient's ABG results reveal $PaCO_2 = 55$ mm Hg. Which of the following changes should be made to the ventilator to reduce the patient's $PaCO_2$ to 40 mm Hg?
   a. Increase the V_T to 620 mL.
   b. Decrease the V_T to 400 mL.
   c. Increase the rate to 18 breaths/min.
   d. Decrease the rate to 10 breaths/min.

6. A patient with a white blood cell count of 13.3×10^3/mcL is coughing up moderate amounts of yellow secretions. Physical examination reveals decreased breath sounds and dullness to percussion. These findings are consistent with which of the following?
   a. Airway trauma
   b. Pulmonary embolism
   c. Pneumonia
   d. Pulmonary edema

7. Which of the following can cause an increase in physiologic dead space?
   1. Pulmonary embolism
   2. An increase in V_T
   3. Low cardiac output
   4. High alveolar pressures
   a. 1 only
   b. 1 and 2
   c. 1, 3, and 4
   d. 1, 2, 3, and 4

8. A patient receiving mechanical ventilation should not be transported under which of the following conditions?
   1. Patient is hemodynamically unstable.
   2. It is not possible to monitor cardiac function.
   3. Patient is nasally intubated.
   4. Patient has multiple IV lines.
   a. 1 only
   b. 1 and 2
   c. 1, 3, and 4
   d. 1, 2, 3, and 4

9. Methods for managing the ventilatory status of a patient with unilateral lung disease include which of the following?
   1. Use of a double-lumen ET
   2. Instillation of normal saline prior to suctioning
   3. Bronchodilator therapy via small volume nebulizer
   4. Position the patient laterally so that the good lung is dependent
   a. 1 only
   b. 1, 2, and 3
   c. 1, 2, 3, and 4
   d. 1 and 4

10. The concept of *patient-centered mechanical ventilation* includes which of the following?
    a. Determining patient comfort level
    b. Maintaining a P_aO_2 greater than 60 mm Hg
    c. Maintaining $P_{plateau}$ less than 40 cm H_2O
    d. Determining nutritional needs

13 Improving Oxygenation and Management of Acute Respiratory Distress Syndrome

LEARNING OBJECTIVES

On completion of this chapter the reader will be able to do the following:

1. Calculate a desired F_IO_2 needed to achieve a desired P_aO_2, based on current ventilator settings and blood gases.
2. Calculate a patient's pulmonary shunt fraction.
3. Identify indications and contraindications for continuous positive airway pressure (CPAP) and positive end-expiratory pressure (PEEP).
4. List the primary goal of PEEP and the conditions in which high levels of PEEP are most often used.
5. From a PEEP study providing arterial blood gases (ABGs) and hemodynamic data, determine the optimal PEEP level.
6. Describe the most appropriate method of establishing an optimal level of PEEP for a patient with acute respiratory distress syndrome (ARDS) using a recruitment-derecruitment maneuver and the deflection point (lower inflection point during deflation or derecruitment).
7. Explain the effects of PEEP/CPAP therapy on a patient with a unilateral lung disease.
8. Describe the problems associated with initiating PEEP in a patient with an untreated pneumothorax.
9. Recommend adjustments in PEEP and ventilator settings based on the physical assessment of the patient, ABGs, and ventilator parameters.
10. Compare static compliance, hemodynamic data, and ABGs as indicators of an optimal PEEP.
11. Identify from patient assessment and ABGs when it is appropriate to change from CPAP to mechanical ventilation with PEEP.
12. Identify the severity of ARDS using the P_aO_2/F_IO_2 ratio.
13. Recommend an appropriate tidal volume (V_T) setting in a patient with ARDS.
14. Identify the maximum $P_{plateau}$ value to use for patients with ARDS.
15. Identify the weaning criteria that should be used to liberate a patient from PEEP or CPAP.
16. Recommend a PEEP setting based on the inflection point on the deflation curve using the pressure-volume (PV) loop for a patient with ARDS.
17. Describe the procedure for prone positioning in ventilated patients with ARDS.
18. List potential problems associated with placing the patient in a prone position during mechanical ventilation.

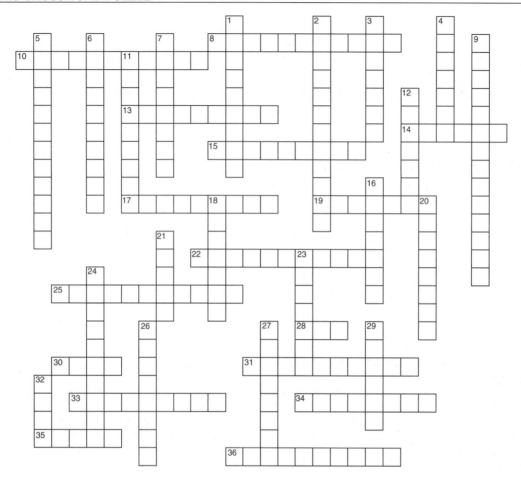

Across

8 Hemorrhaging or dehydration can cause this
10 A maneuver used to open collapsed alveoli
13 The phase of ARDS characterized by inflammation and alveolar filling
14 Lung units
15 Point that occurs when a large number of lung units collapse quickly
17 Zone 3 of the lungs is _____
19 The PEEP level that has maximum benefit
22 Type of pulmonary edema due to congestive heart failure (CHF)
25 Partial or complete collapse of previously expanded areas of lung producing a shrunken, airless state
28 The point on a static pressure-volume curve where the slope of the line changes significantly (abbreviation)
30 _____-billed appearance of pressure-volume curve shows over distention
31 Injury to the lung parenchyma caused by excessive pressures in the lungs
33 _____ alveolitis is the second phase of ARDS
34 Toward the head area
35 Perfusion without ventilation
36 A type of hypoxia caused by cyanide poisoning

Down

1 A type of inflammatory mediator
2 Creates a resistance to gas flow through an orifice (two words)
3 Alter F_IO_2 depending on oxygen saturation
4 Pressure that pulls fluid out of tissues
5 High thoracic pressures can reduce this (two words)
6 Material produced by type II pneumocytes
7 Has blood flowing through its capillaries
9 Keep F_IO_2 low to avoid this (two words)
11 A resistor that maintains pressure independent of flow
12 A pressure measurement taken during positive-pressure ventilation (PPV) after a breath has been delivered to the patient and before exhalation has begun
16 Material that some CPAP masks are made from
18 Type of PV loop obtained during gas flow
20 Chemical that causes inflammation
21 A Drager ventilator
23 A Hamilton ventilator
24 Point that occurs where a large number of lung units collapse quickly
26 Cellular death
27 Breath sound indicative of pulmonary edema
29 Toward the base of the spine
32 A specific clinical disorder that benefits from PEEP (abbreviation)

CHAPTER REVIEW QUESTIONS

1. Explain the difference between hypoxemia and hypoxia.

2. What information does the measurement of oxygen delivery provide?

3. What are the formulas used for calculating oxygen delivery and consumption?

4. How often should the F_IO_2 be monitored on adult and pediatric patients receiving mechanical ventilation?

5. How soon after a change in F_IO_2 is made can an ABG be drawn?

6. At what level should the F_IO_2 be maintained to help prevent the complications of oxygen toxicity?

7. By what mechanism can breathing 100% oxygen contribute to hypoxemia?

8. What is the target range for P_aO_2 when administering supplemental oxygen for most adult patients?

9. Your patient is receiving an F_IO_2 of 0.8 yet their P_aO_2 remains low. What could be happening?

10. What formula is used to calculate the desired F_IO_2 necessary to obtain a desired P_aO_2?

11. Thirty minutes after initiating pressure-targeted ventilation an ABG is drawn with the following results: pH = 7.43, P_aCO_2 = 43 mm Hg, P_aO_2 = 50 mm Hg. The F_IO_2 is set at 75%, with a PEEP level of 5 cm H_2O. What F_IO_2 is needed to achieve a desired P_aO_2 of 60 mm Hg?

12. What is the significance of calculating a patient's pulmonary shunt?

13. What is the classic shunt equation for calculating the patient's pulmonary shunt?

14. Given the following information, calculate the patient's pulmonary shunt fraction : $Cc'O_2$ = 20.4 vol%, CaO_2 = 19.8 vol%, $C'O_2$ = 13.4 vol%

15. Define mean airway pressure ($\bar{P}aw$).

16. List five factors that affect $\bar{P}aw$ during PPV.

    a.
    b.
    c.
    d.
    e.

17. How does increasing $\bar{P}aw$ increase P_aO_2 in the presence of ventilation/perfusion abnormalities and/or diffusion defects?

18. List four methods of increasing $\bar{P}aw$:

    a.
    b.
    c.
    d.

19. What are four goals of PEEP/CPAP therapy?

    a. _____

    b. _____

    c. _____

    d. _____

20. Explain the difference between the terms PEEP and CPAP.

    _____

    _____

    _____

21. How is PEEP applied to the lungs during mechanical ventilation and what is the desired physiologic result?

    _____

    _____

    _____

22. List four devices capable of applying PEEP/CPAP to the airway.

    a. _____

    b. _____

    c. _____

    d. _____

23. List the patient criteria necessary for placing a patient on mask CPAP.

    _____

    _____

    _____

24. List four hazards associated with the use of mask CPAP.

    a. _____

    b. _____

    c. _____

    d. _____

25. List six indications for PEEP therapy.

    a. _____

    b. _____

    c. _____

    d. _____

    e. _____

    f. _____

26. What is the difference between physiologic PEEP and therapeutic PEEP?

    _____

    _____

    _____

    _____

27. What is optimal PEEP?

    _____

    _____

    _____

    _____

28. What physiologic parameters are monitored while determining optimal PEEP?

    _____

    _____

    _____

    _____

29. During volume-controlled ventilation, the PEEP level is set at +5 cm H_2O and the P_{peak} is 42 cm H_2O. After the PEEP is increased to 10 cm H_2O, the P_{peak} is now measured at 48 cm H_2O. Has the patient's condition worsened? What caused the increase in P_{peak}?

    _____

    _____

    _____

30. What happens within the independent zones of lungs with ARDS when PEEP is applied in increasing levels? How can this be avoided?

    _____

    _____

    _____

31. How does positive pressure benefit patients with acute pulmonary edema due to CHF?

    _____

    _____

    _____

32. When PEEP is indicated, how soon should it be initiated? Explain your answer.

    _____

    _____

33. List three specific clinical disorders that may benefit from the use of PEEP/CPAP.

    a. _____

    b. _____

    c. _____

34. What effects will PEEP have on a patient with an untreated pneumothorax?

    _____

    _____

    _____

35. Why is PEEP therapy not always beneficial to patients with emphysema?

    _____

    _____

36. List five criteria that may indicate that a patient is ready for a trial reduction of PEEP.

    a. _____

    b. _____

    c. _____

    d. _____

    e. _____

37. Define ARDS.

    _____

    _____

    _____

38. What onset of time does the *Berlin Definition* of ARDS specify?

    _____

39. Identify the two phases of ARDS and the characteristics of each.

    a. _____

    b. _____

40. Why does pulmonary edema develop in the ARDS patient?

    a. _____

    b. _____

41. How should fluid be managed in the ARDS patient?

    _____

42. What are the two categories of ARDS?

    a. _____

    b. _____

43. Define the following terms related to the computed tomography in an ARDS patient.

    a. Ground glass opacification: _____

    b. Consolidation: _____

    c. Reticular pattern: _____

44. What are the basic points that should be kept in mind when managing ventilated patients with ARDS using an open-lung or lung-protective strategy?

    a. _____

    b. _____

    c. _____

    d. _____

    e. _____

    f. _____

    g. _____

45. Explain how a normal lung can become damaged during the management of ARDS.

    _____

46. What is the purpose of performing a slow or static PV loop?

    _____

    _____

    _____

47. How is the inflation portion of the PV loop utilized?

    _____

    _____

    _____

48. Once the deflation point of the PV loop is identified, what happens?

    _____

    _____

49. What is the difference between a static PV loop and a quasi-static PV loop?

    _____

    _____

50. A lung recruitment maneuver provides the following information: lower inflection point (LIP) is 10 cm H_2O, upper inflection point on the inspiratory limb (UIPi) is 20 cm H_2O, and the upper inflection point on the deflation portion of the curve (UIPd) is 5 cm H_2O. What should the PEEP be set at and why?

_____

_____

_____

51. To avoid overdistention in the patient from the previous question, peak inspiratory pressure (PIP) should not exceed what pressure?

_____

52. Give three examples of types of lung recruitment maneuvers.

a. _____

b. _____

c. _____

53. An ARDS patient is on pressure-controlled continuous mandatory ventilation at a rate of 10 breaths/min; inspiratory-to-expiratory ratio 1:1, PC is set at 20 cm H_2O above PEEP, and PEEP is 10 cm H_2O. Describe how manipulating the PEEP level may be used to establish an optimal PEEP level for this patient.

_____

_____

_____

_____

_____

_____

_____

Use the following table to answer Questions 54 and 55.

Time	0800	0805	0810	0815	0820	0825	0830	0835	0840	0845
PEEP (cm H_2O)	0	5	10	15	20	25	30	35	40	35
C_s (mL/cm H_2O)	27	27	27	29	32	36	38	41	40	40

Time	0850	0855	0900	0905	0910	0915	0920	0925	0930	0935
PEEP (cm H_2O)	32.5	30	27.5	25	22.5	20	17.5	15	12.5	10
C_s (mL/cm H_2O)	40	38	38	38	38	37	37	28	28	27

54. At what time, PEEP level, and Cs did the UIPd point occur?

_____

55. What is the appropriate PEEP setting for this patient?

_____

56. List two reasons for placing an ARDS patient in the prone position.

a. _____

b. _____

57. List the six mechanisms believed to improve oxygenation with prone positioning in the ARDS patient.

a. _____

b. _____

c. _____

d. _____

e. _____

f. _____

58. What should be the first thing done before placing a patient in the prone position?

_____

59. What is the absolute contraindication to prone positioning?

_____

60. Describe the two methods used to manage the ventilatory status of patients with unilateral lung disease.

a. _____

b. _____

CRITICAL THINKING QUESTIONS

1. Use the following PV loop to answer Questions a through c.

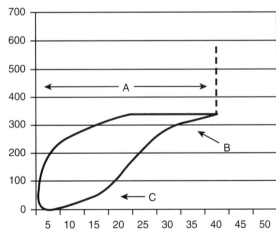

a. Identify the following points in the pressure-volume curve.

Point A _____

Point B _____

Point C _____

b. Identify the point at which the lungs are overstretched.

_____

_____

c. Identify the point that may correlate with an increase in $PaCO_2$.

_____

_____

_____

2. The following volume-pressure curve was obtained from a patient receiving volume-controlled ventilation.

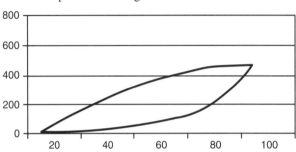

a. What is the approximate PIP?

_____

b. What is the approximate exhaled V_T?

_____

c. By observing this volume-pressure curve, can it be determined whether the high airway pressure was caused by a decrease in compliance or by an increase in airway resistance?

_____

3. A patient with ARDS and refractory hypoxemia is being ventilated in a pressure-control mode. The physician would like to perform a recruitment maneuver with increased PEEP. Can you explain the process to the physician's medical student who is asking how it works?

_____

_____

_____

Case Study 1

A 38-year-old patient is admitted to the emergency department and placed on volume-controlled mechanical ventilation for aspiration pneumonia. A postintubation radiograph reveals that the endotracheal tube is in proper position. There is complete opacification of the right lung. The left lung appears normal. The PIP 62 cm H_2O, and $P_{plateau}$ 55 cm H_2O. Ventilator settings and ABG results are as follows:

Mode	VC-CMV	pH	7.43
F_IO_2	1.0	$PaCO_2$	38 mm Hg
Frequency	20	P_aO_2	40 mm Hg
V_T	800 mL	HCO_3^-	23 mEq/L
PEEP	15 cm H_2O	BE	0 mEq/L

1. What could be causing the severe hypoxemia?

_____

_____

2. What should the therapist recommend?

_____

_____

Case Study 2

A 26-year-old male is 5 feet 6 inches tall and weighs 56.8 kg (125 lb). He was admitted for a heroin overdose, and was intubated and placed on volume-controlled ventilation. Chest radiograph reveals bilateral "fluffy" infiltrates. Ventilatory data and ABGs are as follows:

Mode	VC-CMV	pH	7.37
F_IO_2	1.0	$PaCO_2$	43 mm Hg
Frequency	12	P_aO_2	44 mm Hg
V_T	600 mL	S_aO_2	85%
PEEP	5 cm H_2O	HCO_3^-	23 mEq/L
PIP	55 cm H_2O	BE	0 mEq/L
$P_{plateau}$	48 cm H_2O		

1. Interpret the ABG.

_____

2. What is the significance of the $P_{plateau}$?

_____

_____

3. What should the therapist recommend to treat the hypoxemia and high ventilating pressures?

_____

_____

NBRC-STYLE QUESTIONS

1. By what mechanism does PEEP cause an increase in intracranial pressure?
   a. Cardiac output and venous return are increased.
   b. Stroke volume is decreased.
   c. There is an increase in central venous pressure.
   d. Venous return is decreased, which results in intracranial hemorrhage.

2. Which of the following is an absolute contraindication to the use of PEEP or CPAP therapy?
   a. Increased intracranial pressure
   b. Severe hyperventilation
   c. Decreased lung compliance
   d. Untreated pneumothorax or tension pneumothorax

3. A 35-year-old patient diagnosed with ARDS is receiving pressure-controlled mechanical ventilation. Based on ABG results, the PEEP is increased from 14 to 18 cm H_2O. Which of the following should the therapist monitor immediately after making the change?
   a. Cardiac output
   b. Pulse oximetry
   c. Hemoglobin
   d. Serum potassium

4. If the total arterial content of oxygen (CaO_2) is 16.94 vol%, and the cardiac output is 12.54 L/min, how much oxygen is being delivered?
   a. 1000 mL/min
   b. 2.124 L/min
   c. 3.450 L/min
   d. 3.926 L/min

5. Which of the following is the primary mechanism by which PEEP increases P_aO_2 and improves compliance?
   a. Reduction in mean airway pressure
   b. Increase in minute ventilation
   c. Recruitment of collapsed alveoli
   d. Decrease in cardiac output

6. What effect does PEEP have on both P_aO_2 and $PaCO_2$?
   a. Both P_aO_2 and $PaCO_2$ and should increase.
   b. P_aO_2 should increase and $PaCO_2$ should decrease.
   c. Both P_aO_2 and $PaCO_2$ and should decrease.
   d. $PaCO_2$ should remain unaffected and P_aO_2 should increase.

7. Which of the following is a direct lung insult that can result in ARDS?
   1. Pneumonia
   2. Aspiration
   3. Sepsis
   4. Smoke inhalation
   a. 1 only
   b. 1 and 2
   c. 1, 2, and 4
   d. 1, 2, 3, and 4

8. Which of the following conditions is a potential complication when instituting PEEP therapy?
   1. Decrease in cardiac output
   2. Barotrauma
   3. Altered cardiac function
   4. Decrease in urine output
   a. 1 only
   b. 3 and 4
   c. 1, 3 and 4
   d. 1, 2, 3, and 4

9. What could be the most likely cause of an increased $PaCO_2$ after an increase in the level of PEEP?
   a. Tension pneumothorax
   b. Lung overdistention
   c. An increase in compliance
   d. A decrease in airway resistance

10. When managing a patient with ARDS receiving mechanical ventilation and PEEP, what can be done to help alleviate the problem of excessive lung water?
    a. Ventilate with large tidal volumes.
    b. Increase the amount of intravenous fluids.
    c. Patients should be placed on diuretic therapy.
    d. Keep PIPs below 50 cm H_2O.

Ventilator-Associated Pneumonia

LEARNING OBJECTIVES

Upon completion of this chapter the reader will be able to do the following:

1. Define *ventilator-associated pneumonia* (VAP) and *hospital-acquired pneumonia* (HAP).
2. Differentiate between early-onset VAP and late-onset VAP and describe the overall incidence of VAP.
3. Discuss the prognosis, including morbidity and mortality rates, for patients diagnosed with VAP.
4. Identify the most common pathogenic microorganisms associated with VAP.
5. List nonpharmacologic and pharmacologic therapeutic interventions that have been shown to increase the risk of development of VAP.
6. Describe the sequence of events that are typically associated with the pathogenesis of VAP.
7. Discuss the advantages and disadvantages of using clinical findings versus quantitative diagnostic techniques to identify patients with VAP.
8. Briefly describe the criteria for starting empiric antibiotic therapy for patients without evidence of multidrug-resistant (MDR) infections and for those patients with risk of developing MDR infections.
9. Define *deescalation of antibiotic therapy* and how it can be used to reduce the emergence of MDR pathogens.
10. Discuss how *ventilator bundles* can be used to prevent VAP and the emergence of MDR pathogens in the clinical setting.

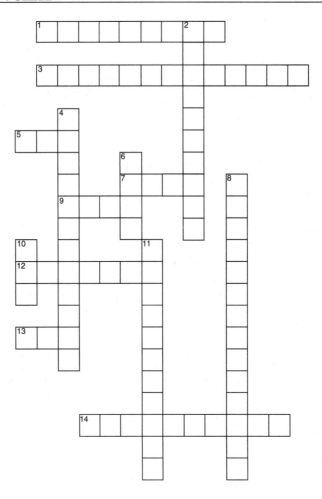

Across

1 VAP that develops later than 72 hours following tracheal intubation (two words)
3 Infection by multiple pathogenic microorganisms
5 Pathogens resistant to certain antibiotics (abbreviation)
7 A major complication of VAP
9 An assessment criteria including fever, leukocyte count, tracheal secretion characteristics, and oxygenation status
12 Guidelines for the management of adults with HAP, VAP, and health care–associated pneumonia (abbreviation)
13 Pneumonia that develops 48 hours after a patient has been placed on mechanical ventilation (abbreviation)
14 Infection acquired in the health care setting

Down

2 VAP that develops between 48 and 72 hours after tracheal intubation (two words)
4 Used to obtain cultures from the lower respiratory tract
6 Continuous aspiration of subglottic secretions
8 Prolonged antibiotic used for intensive care unit (ICU) patients may favor selection with resistant organisms responsible for this (two words)
10 Bronchial alveolar lavage (abbreviation)
11 Common respiratory infection seen in patients with cystic fibrosis (abbreviation)

CHAPTER REVIEW QUESTIONS

1. VAP is most often caused by what type of infection?

   _____

2. What are the two classifications of VAP? Describe the differences.

   a. _____

   b. _____

3. What are some common gram-negative anaerobes isolated from nosocomial pneumonias?

   _____

   _____

   _____

4. List two common gram-positive aerobes isolated from nosocomial pneumonias?

   a. _____

   b. _____

5. What is the mortality rate range caused by VAP?

   _____

6. Guidelines for the management of patients with VAP focus on

   _____

   _____

   _____

7. What is one of the most common nosocomial infection encountered in the ICU?

   _____

8. The incidence of VAP for all intubated patients ranges between what percentages?

   _____

9. List five causes of VAP.

   a. _____

   b. _____

   c. _____

   d. _____

   e. _____

10. List 10 host-related factors that may increase the development of VAP in a patient.

    a. _____

    b. _____

    c. _____

    d. _____

    e. _____

    f. _____

    g. _____

    h. _____

    i. _____

    j. _____

11. What types of patients are typically at highest risk for the development of VAP?

    _____

12. Mechanically Ventilated patients with chronic obstructive pulmonary disease (COPD) are susceptible to what VAP-causing pathogens?

    _____

    _____

    _____

13. Mechanically Ventilated patients with cystic fibrosis are more susceptible to what VAP-causing pathogens?

    _____

    _____

14. VAP is a major complication of and increases the mortality rate for patients with what respiratory condition?

    _____

15. List four common risk factors for the development of MDR infections.

    a. _____

    b. _____

    c. _____

    d. _____

16. List six nonpharmacologic interventions that are associated with the increased risk of VAP.

   a. _____

   b. _____

   c. _____

   d. _____

   e. _____

   f. _____

17. List four pharmacologic interventions that can lead to the development of VAP.

   a. _____

   b. _____

   c. _____

   d. _____

18. Describe briefly the sequence of events that lead to VAP.

   _____

   _____

19. What are the six clinical assessments of the Clinical Pulmonary Infection Score (CPIS) criteria?

   a. _____

   b. _____

   c. _____

   d. _____

   e. _____

   f. _____

20. What happens to the oropharyngeal flora of invasively ventilated, critically ill patients?

   _____

21. When using all six criteria of the CPIS, what score indicates evidence of the presence of VAP?

   _____

22. What procedure has been shown to significantly improve the diagnosis of VAP?

   _____

23. What is the difference between clinical assessment (qualitative) and quantitative diagnosis of VAP?

   _____

24. The most important nonpharmacologic prevention strategy to reduce the risk of clinicians transmitting infectious microorganisms from one patient to another is what?

   _____

25. What are some ways to reduce aspiration of gastric contents?

   _____

   _____

   _____

26. What is a common pathogen associated with percutaneous tracheostomy?

   _____

27. To lessen the risk of VAP, when should ventilator circuits be changed?

   _____

   _____

28. List four pharmacologic interventions to help reduce the risk of VAP.

   a. _____

   b. _____

   c. _____

   d. _____

29. List four quantitative techniques used to diagnose VAP.

   a. _____

   b. _____

   c. _____

   d. _____

30. Successful treatment of VAP requires what two types of assessments?

   a. _____

   b. _____

31. What position should a ventilated patient be in to reduce the incidence of aspiration?

_____

32. Why does oral intubation pose less of a risk for VAP than nasal intubation?

_____

33. Pharmacologic and nonpharmacologic strategies to reduce the incidence of VAP are incorporated into evidence-based practices known as

_____

CRITICAL THINKING QUESTIONS

1. A 69-year-old male patient with a history of COPD is intubated and is receiving mechanical ventilation because of trauma sustained in a motor vehicle collision. What are some factors that put this patient at an increased risk for developing VAP and what can the therapist do to reduce this risk?

_____

_____

_____

_____

2. Why is a patient's past medical history important when determining antibiotic therapy?

_____

CASE STUDIES

Case Study

A patient with a history of cystic fibrosis develops a fever with purulent tracheobronchial secretions 4 days after endotracheal intubation and mechanical ventilation. The respiratory therapist suspects VAP.

1. What type of VAP is likely?

_____

2. Considering the patient's past medical history, what is the most likely pathogen causing the pneumonia?

_____

3. What can be done to diagnosis the pathogen?

_____

NBRC-STYLE QUESTIONS

1. VAP is most commonly caused by which of the following?
   a. Viral infection
   b. Fungal infection
   c. Bacterial infection
   d. Acute respiratory distress syndrome

2. With regard to VAP, COPD patients are at increased risk from which of the following pathogenic organisms?
   a. *Haemophilus influenzae*
   b. *Candida albicans*
   c. *Klebsiella pneumoniae*
   d. *Pseudomonas aeruginosa*

3. Therapeutic interventions that can lead to the development of VAP include which of the following?
   a. Inappropriate antimicrobial therapy
   b. Frequent arterial blood gas analysis
   c. Noninvasive ventilation
   d. Semirecumbent positioning of the patient

4. Which of the following falls in the category of ventilator-associated event as defined by the Centers for Disease Control and Prevention?
   1. VAP
   2. Ventilator-associated condition
   3. Infection-related ventilator-associated complication
   4. Acute respiratory distress syndrome
   a. 1 and 3 only
   b. 1 and 2 only
   c. 1, 2, and 3 only
   d. 1, 2, 3, and 4

5. What is the nonpharmacologic intervention most associated with VAP?
   a. Frequent changing of the ventilator circuit
   b. Use of an endotracheal tube or tracheostomy during mechanical ventilation
   c. Use of bronchoscopes
   d. Reusable ventilator probes

6. During critical illness, the shift in the normal flora of the oropharyngeal tract to gram-negative bacilli and *Staphylococcus aureus* may be due to which of the following factors?
   1. Comorbidities
   2. Malnutrition
   3. Decreased airway pH
   4. Decreased production of proteases
   a. 1 and 3 only
   b. 1 and 2 only
   c. 3 and 4 only
   d. 2 and 4 only

139

7. Inappropriate use of what intervention is associated with the emergence of MDR pathogens?
   a. Noninvasive positive-pressure ventilation
   b. Antibiotics
   c. Tracheostomy tubes
   d. Fiberoptic bronchoscopy

8. Which of the following refers to the process of focusing the types and duration of antibiotics used to treat VAP?
   a. Broad-spectrum antibiotic therapy
   b. Ventilator bundles
   c. Nonpharmacologic interventions
   d. Deescalating antibiotic therapy

9. What is a benefit of the use of mini bronchoalveolar lavage as a nonbronchoscopic technique?
   a. It is less expensive than bronchoscopy
   b. It is commonly performed by a pulmonologist
   c. Accuracy of sampling location within the lung
   d. Direct visualization of the sampling site can be obtained

10. Strategies to prevent VAP include:
    a. Ventilator bundles
    b. Placing all patients in strict isolation
    c. Reduce the patients receiving mechanical ventilation
    d. Limit intubations and focus patient care on the use of continuous positive airway pressure

15 Sedatives, Analgesics, and Paralytics

On completion of this chapter the reader will be able to do the following:

1. List the most common sedatives and analgesics used in the treatment of critically ill patients.
2. Discuss the indications, contraindications, and potential side effects of each of the sedatives and analgesic agents reviewed.
3. Describe the most common method of assessing the need for and level of sedation.
4. Describe the Ramsay Scale.
5. Discuss the advantages and disadvantages of using benzodiazepines, neuroleptics, anesthetic agents, and opioids in the management of mechanically ventilated patients.
6. Discuss the mode of action of depolarizing and nondepolarizing paralytics.
7. Explain how the train-of-four method (TOF) is used to assess the level of paralysis in critically ill patients.
8. Contrast the indications, contraindications, and potential side effects associated with using various types of neuromuscular blocking agents (NMBAs).
9. Recommend a medication for a mechanically ventilated patient with severe anxiety and agitation.

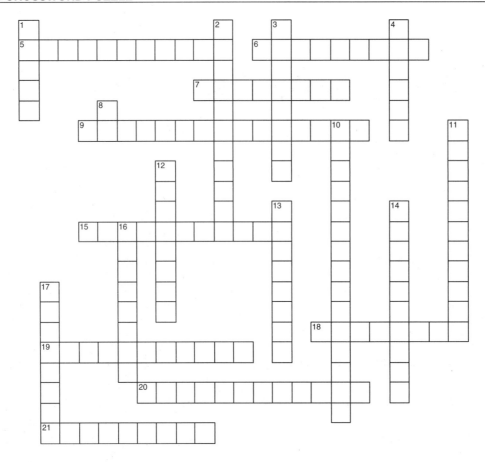

Across

5 Type of amnesia in which the acquisition and encoding of new information that can potentially lead to memories of unpleasant experiences prevented

6 Facilitates invasive procedures by preventing movement

7 An anesthetic agent common in the intensive care unit (ICU)

9 A depolarizing neuromuscular blocking agent

15 A graduated single-category scale that is used to assess the level of sedation (two words)

18 A benzodiazepine drug

19 Method of monitoring the depth of paralysis with an electrical current (three words)

20 An agent that causes skeletal muscle paralysis by causing a reversal of the resting membrane potential in excitable cell membranes

21 Drug of choice for sedating mechanically ventilated patients for longer than 24 hours, which generally produces only minimal effects on cardiovascular function

Down

1 An opioid receptor that mediates the sedative effects

2 Haloperidol is included in this category of drugs

3 An opioid antagonist

4 Pinpoint pupils

8 An opioid receptor that is responsible for analgesia

10 Agent that inhibits the action of acetylcholine at the neuromuscular junction

11 A nondepolarizing NMBA

12 Agent that reduces anxiety and agitation and promotes sleep

13 Disorganized thought patterns and excessive, nonpurposeful motor activity

14 Reverses the effects of benzodiazepines

16 A naturally occurring opioid

17 A synthetic opioid that is approximately 100 to 150 times more potent than morphine

Chapter **15** **Sedatives, Analgesics, and Paralytics**

CHAPTER REVIEW QUESTIONS

1. What effects do sedatives have on the body?

_____

2. Describe a clinical situation when paralysis may be indicated during mechanical ventilation.

_____

3. List the four types of pharmacologic agents commonly used for sedation in the ICU. Give at least one example of each.

   a. _____

   b. _____

   c. _____

   d. _____

4. List and define the four Joint Commission–defined levels of sedation.

   a. _____

   b. _____

   c. _____

   d. _____

5. What level of sedation may be necessary when a patient's breathing is asynchronous with the mechanical ventilatory mode?

_____

6. What level of sedation is necessary during weaning from mechanical ventilation?

_____

7. What scoring systems may be used to assess the level of sedation in adults and children?

_____

Use the Scoring System in Table 15-1 to answer Questions 8 through 10.

TABLE 15-1   The Ramsay Sedation Scale

Score	Description
1	Patient is awake but anxious, agitated, and restless.
2	Patient is awake, cooperative, oriented, and tranquil.
3	Patient is semi-asleep but responds to verbal commands.
4	Patient is asleep and has a brisk response to a light glabellar tap or loud auditory stimulus.
5	Patient is asleep and has a sluggish response to a light glabellar tap or loud auditory stimulus.
6	Patient is asleep and has no response to a light glabellar tap or loud auditory stimulus.

Chapter **15 Sedatives, Analgesics, and Paralytics**

8. What range of scores indicates adequate sedation?

_____

9. What score indicates the need for sedation?

_____

10. What scores indicate oversedation of a patient?

_____

11. Why are benzodiazepines the drugs of choice for the treatment of anxiety in critical care?

_____

_____

12. Explain the mode of action for benzodiazepines.

_____

_____

_____

_____

13. List three factors that can alter the intensity and duration of action of various benzodiazepines.

   a. _____

   b. _____

   c. _____

14. Describe a pathologic process that can prolong recovery from treatment with benzodiazepines.

_____

15. Why does diazepam have a rapid onset of action?

_____

_____

_____

16. How is diazepam administered in the ICU setting?

_____

_____

17. Acutely agitated patients are best treated with which benzodiazepine? Why?

_____

_____

18. How can prolonged sedation occur with midazolam?

_____

_____

_____

144

19. Which benzodiazepine is best suited for sedating mechanically ventilated patients in the ICU for longer than 24 hours?

_____

20. You are the respiratory therapist working in the emergency department of a busy hospital. A patient is brought in who was found unresponsive with an empty bottle of Valium near him. What medication would you suggest to reverse the drug? Are there any side effects that you would be concerned about following its administration?

_____

21. Potential side effects of continual use of lorazepam (Ativan) include the following:

    a. _____

    b. _____

    c. _____

22. What class of drugs is routinely used to treat extremely agitated and delirious patients in the ICU?

_____

23. The drug most often used to treat ICU delirium is _____.

24. List three of the side effects of the drug in the Question 23.

    a. _____

    b. _____

    c. _____

25. List the hemodynamic effects of propofol.

_____

_____

26. What are the advantages and disadvantages of using propofol drug to sedate neurologic patients?

Disadvantages	Advantages
_____	_____
_____	_____
_____	_____
_____	_____
_____	_____
_____	_____

27. List the two opioids most commonly used in the ICU setting.

    a. _____

    b. _____

28. List three effects that opiates have on the body.

a. _____

b. _____

c. _____

29. List 10 side effects of opioids.

a. _____

b. _____

c. _____

d. _____

e. _____

f. _____

g. _____

h. _____

i. _____

j. _____

30. What determines the severity of the side effects of opioids?

_____

31. Which drug can reverse the respiratory depression caused by opioids?

_____

32. What effects does morphine have on the central nervous system?

_____

_____

_____

33. How does morphine affect the gastrointestinal tract?

_____

_____

_____

_____

34. How does morphine affect the cardiovascular system?

_____

_____

35. Which opioid should be used for a patient who is hemodynamically unstable?

_____

36. Increased intracranial pressure caused by traumatic brain injury may be controlled by a combination of which two drugs?

_____

37. What is the difference between depolarizing and nondepolarizing agents?

_____

38. List four clinical situations that may require NMBAs to be used while a patient is being mechanically ventilated.

a. _____

b. _____

c. _____

d. _____

39. What is the purpose of TOF?

_____

40. Describe how TOF works.

_____

_____

41. According to the Society for Critical Care Medicine, what indicates that an adequate amount of NMBA is being administered when TOF is used?

_____

42. What other medication is necessary when a paralytic agent is used?

_____

_____

43. The most widely used NMBA for facilitating endotracheal intubation is

_____

Its onset of action and duration of action is

_____

44. What are the most common side effects of the drug referred to in Question 43?

_____

_____

_____

_____

45. Which nondepolarizing NMBA has the longest duration of action?

_____

46. Which nondepolarizing NMBAs are used for intermediate duration?

_____

_____

47. What type of patient could experience prolonged paralysis after discontinuation of pancuronium? Why?

_____

_____

_____

_____

48. Seizures have been associated with which nondepolarizing NMBA?

_____

49. Mast cell degranulation and histamine release, which may lead to peripheral vasodilation and hypotension, are associated with which nondepolarizing NMBA?

_____

50. Which nondepolarizing NMBAs are ideal for patients with renal and hepatic insufficiency?

_____

51. The nondepolarizing NMBA of choice for patients who are hemodynamically unstable, have cardiac disease, or are at risk of histamine release is

_____.

52. List two side effects of the long-term use of NMBAs.

a. _____

b. _____

CRITICAL THINKING QUESTIONS

1. When an NMBA is administered to a patient receiving ventilatory care, what ventilator alarms should be activated?

_____

_____

_____

2. Which type of opioid is best suited to a patient who has asthma? Why?

_____

_____

_____

_____

CASE STUDIES

Case Study

The respiratory therapist checks on an ICU patient receiving ventilatory support with ventilator-controlled synchronized mandatory ventilation (VC-SIMV). The ventilator settings are as follows: rate = 6 breaths/min, V_T = 600 mL, F_IO_2 = 0.4, positive end-expiratory pressure = 5 cm H_2O. The mode was change to VC-IMV 1 hour ago because of dyssynchrony. The patient's legs are hanging over the bed railing, and his hands are on the ventilator tubing. The high-pressure alarm is activating with every breath at a rate of 35 breaths/min. The patient is anxious and uncooperative and remains dyssynchronous with the ventilator despite adjustments made to the ventilator settings.

1. What would be the most appropriate type of medication to deliver at this time?

_____

2. What concerns should the respiratory therapist have about the patient's ventilator settings?

_____

_____

_____

_____

1. Which of the following drugs can be used to reverse the effects of benzodiazepines?
   a. Pseudocholinesterase
   b. Flumazenil (Romazicon)
   c. Fentanyl citrate (Sublimaze)
   d. Naloxone (Narcan)

2. The respiratory therapist is called to the postanesthesia care unit to assist in the weaning of a postoperative patient who had a cholecystectomy. The patient is 3 hours postop and is still apneic and receiving full ventilatory support. The medication(s) that could be used to facilitate ventilator weaning is (are) which of the following?
   1. Naloxone (Narcan)
   2. Propofol (Diprivan)
   3. Midazolam (Versed)
   4. Flumazenil (Romazicon)
   a. 1 and 4 only
   b. 2 and 4 only
   c. 1 and 3 only
   d. 2 and 3 only

3. An adult patient is in pain, panicky, and fighting the ventilator. The most appropriate medication to control this patient during mechanical ventilation is which of the following?
   a. Propofol (Diprivan)
   b. Haloperidol (Haldol)
   c. Fentanyl citrate (Sublimaze)
   d. Succinylcholine (Anectine)

4. Which of the following is a fast-acting NMBA that is often used to facilitate intubation?
   a. Vecuronium (Norcuron)
   b. Pancuronium (Pavulon)
   c. Midazolam (Versed)
   d. Succinylcholine chloride (Anectine)

5. A mechanically ventilated patient who is hemodynamically unstable needs to be placed on pressure control inverse ratio ventilation and will require paralysis. The most appropriate drug combination for this patient is which of the following?
   a. Succinylcholine chloride (Anectine) and morphine
   b. Propofol (Diprivan) and fentanyl (Sublimaze)
   c. Atracurium besylate (Tracrium) and midazolam (Versed)
   d. Cisatracurium besylate (Nimbex) and flumazenil (Romazicon)

6. A patient with which of the following Ramsay scores is most likely to wean successfully from mechanical ventilation?
   a. 1
   b. 2
   c. 4
   d. 6

7. The depth of paralysis during neuromuscular blockade may be assessed with which of the following?
   a. Ramsay Scale
   b. Serum GABA levels
   c. TOF monitoring
   d. Level of sedation assessment

8. The NMBA that causes histamine release is which of the following?
   a. Atracurium
   b. Cisatracurium
   c. Vecuronium
   d. Pancuronium

9. The NMBA most appropriate for facilitating emergency intubation is which of the following?
   a. Pancuronium (Pavulon)
   b. Vecuronium (Norcuron)
   c. Atracurium (Tracrium)
   d. Succinylcholine chloride (Anectine)

10. The NMBA that can be used in patients with renal or hepatic insufficiency without producing prolonged paralysis is which of the following?
    a. Cisatracurium (Nimbex)
    b. Vecuronium (Norcuron)
    c. Pancuronium (Pavulon)
    d. Succinylcholine chloride (Anectine)

16 Extrapulmonary Effects of Mechanical Ventilation

LEARNING OBJECTIVES

On completion of this chapter the reader will be able to do the following:

1. Explain the effects of positive-pressure ventilation (PPV) on cardiac output and venous return to the heart.
2. Discuss the three factors that can influence cardiac output during PPV.
3. Explain the effects of PPV on gas distribution and pulmonary blood flow in the lungs.
4. Describe how PPV increases intracranial pressure (ICP).
5. Summarize the effects of PPV on renal and endocrine function.
6. Describe the effects of abnormal arterial blood gases on renal function.
7. Name five ways of assessing a patient's nutritional status.
8. Describe techniques that can be used to reduce some of the complications associated with mechanical ventilation.

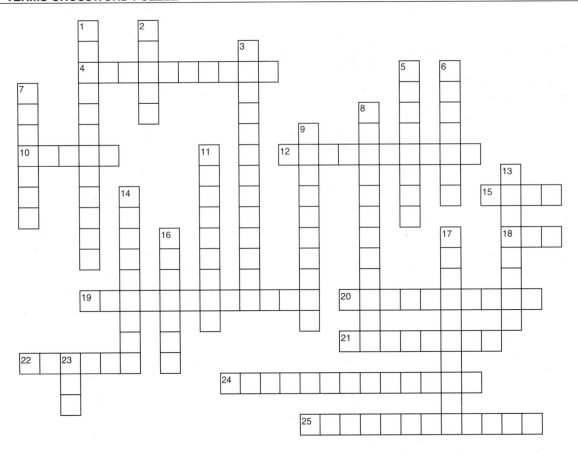

Across

4 This pressure is increased by an inflation hold (two words)
10 Gas always follows the path of _____ resistance
12 Spontaneous inspiration increases blood flow to this structure (two words)
15 18 across plus ICP equals this (abbreviation)
18 The amount of blood flowing to the brain is determined by this (abbreviation)
19 A reduction in this decreases preload to the heart (two words)
20 Through the wall of an organ
21 Antidiuretic hormone release results in this
22 The volume pumped out of a ventricle with one beat
24 This maneuver will increase inspiratory time (two words)
25 Inflammation of many nerves simultaneously

Down

1 A mechanism that maintains blood pressure (BP) in normal individuals receiving PPV
2 A function that can be altered by mechanical ventilation
3 This may decrease with the use of PPV (two words)
5 Reduction in blood flow or supply of oxygenated blood to an organ
6 The structural and functional unit of the kidney
7 Reductions in 19 across decrease this
8 This pressure falls with spontaneous inspiration
9 A drug used to avoid gastrointestinal bleeding
11 When an alveolus is overfilled, this capillary becomes thin
13 A reflex that is blocked by 25 across
14 Compression of the heart
16 The vein that is visible when central venous pressure (CVP) is elevated
17 Urinary output will decrease when this capillary pressure decreases below 75 mm Hg
23 Measuring this provides information about a patient's daily caloric requirements (abbreviation)

CHAPTER REVIEW QUESTIONS

1. List the five bodily functions that PPV can significantly alter.

   a. _____   d. _____

   b. _____   e. _____

   c. _____

2. The physiologic effects of PPV on the cardiovascular system depend on what two factors?

   _____

3. Explain how spontaneous inspiration facilitates venous return to the right heart.

   _____

   _____

   _____

4. During what part of a spontaneous breath is right ventricular preload increased? Why?

   _____

   _____

5. During what part of a spontaneous breath is left ventricular preload decreased? Why?

   _____

   _____

   _____

6. An increase in CVP will do what to the pressure gradient between systemic veins and the right heart?

   _____

Questions 7 through 9 refer to the following figure.

Point Y1
Pressure = 1 cm H_2O

Point Y2
Pressure = 3 cm H_2O

Point Y3
Pressure = 4.5 cm H_2O

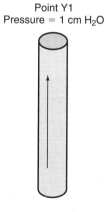
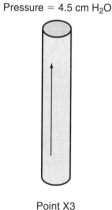

Point X1
Pressure = 5 cm H_2O

Point X2
Pressure = 5 cm H_2O

Point X3
Pressure = 5 cm H_2O

A

B

C

7. Which diagram represents the largest pressure gradient? _____

8. Which diagram represents the smallest pressure gradient? _____

Chapter **16** **Extrapulmonary Effects of Mechanical Ventilation**

9. If each tube in the figure represented the inferior vena cava, the "X" points represented systemic pressure, and the "Y" points represented CVP, which diagram would have the most venous return?

_____

10. What effect does alveolar overdistention have on the pulmonary capillaries and right ventricular afterload?

_____

_____

_____

_____

11. What conditions need to exist for the interventricular septum to move to the left during PPV?

_____

12. How can PPV cause myocardial ischemia?

_____

_____

_____

_____

13. List the compensatory mechanisms responsible for the maintenance of systemic BP during the ventilation of normal individuals.

a. _____

b. _____

c. _____

d. _____

14. List four factors that can block the body's compensatory mechanisms for maintaining arterial BP while a patient is receiving PPV.

a. _____

b. _____

c. _____

d. _____

15. How can a respiratory therapist check that normal vascular reflexes are intact when PPV is being initiated?

_____

16. Normovolemic patients may experience decreases in cardiac output when positive end-expiratory pressure

(PEEP) levels of _____ are used.

17. List the three factors can influence cardiac output during PPV.

a. _____

b. _____

c. _____

18. Explain how PPV can benefit the cardiac function of a patient with left ventricular dysfunction.

_____

_____

19. What pressure exerts the most influence on the extent of harmful effects caused by PPV?

_____

20. Calculate the mean airway pressure using the following parameters: peak inspiratory pressure (PIP) is 25 cm H_2O, T_I is 1 second, and respiratory rate is 12 breaths/min.

_____

_____

_____

_____

21. Add a 1-second inspiratory hold to the previous parameters from question 20 and calculate the mean airway pressure.

_____

_____

_____

_____

22. What happens to the mean airway pressure when an inspiratory hold is added?

_____

23. Calculate the mean airway pressure using the following parameters: PIP is 35 cm H_2O, PEEP is 10 cm H_2O, T_I is 1 second, and respiratory rate is 12 breaths/min. (Notice the ΔP is the same as the PIP in the previous examples.)

_____

_____

_____

_____

_____

24. Calculate the mean airway pressure using the same parameters as in the previous example but add a 1-second inspiratory hold.

_____

_____

_____

_____

_____

25. What type of inspiratory flow produces uneven ventilation?

_____

26. List an inspiratory-to-expiratory ratio that is most likely to cause air trapping and significant hemodynamic complications.

_____

27. What type of T_E allows for better alveolar emptying and less chance of developing intrinsic PEEP?

_____

28. The amount of mean airway pressure required to achieve a certain level of oxygenation may indicate

_____.

29. List five factors that influence mean airway pressure during mechanical ventilation.

a. _____

b. _____

c. _____

d. _____

e. _____

30. Explain why rapid inspiratory flow rates may produce lower mean airway pressures in patients with normal conducting airways.

_____

_____

31. For PEEP levels to affect cardiac output, what circumstances have to exist?

_____

_____

_____

32. In what circumstance would high levels of PEEP *not* cause a decrease in cardiac output?

_____

_____

_____

33. What is the cerebral perfusion pressure when the ICP is 18 cm H_2O and the mean systemic arterial BP is 85 cm H_2O?

_____

34. How can PPV increase ICP?

_____

_____

_____

_____

35. How can an increased ICP be observed clinically?

_____

36. What effect does hyperventilation have on cerebral vessels?

_____

37. List three ways renal function can be altered by PPV?

a. _____

b. _____

c. _____

38. At what glomerular capillary pressure will urinary output become severely reduced?

_____

_____

39. What happens to kidney function when blood flow to the outer cortex decreases and flow to the inner cortex and outer medullary tissue increases?

_____

_____

40. List the three hormones that are involved in fluid and electrolyte balance during PPV and what effects each of these hormones exert.

a. _____

b. _____

c. _____

41. Describe the effects of abnormal arterial blood gases on renal function.

_____

_____

_____

_____

42. What effects does PPV have on the pharmokinetics of certain drugs?

_____

_____

_____

43. How can PPV and PEEP affect liver function?

_____

_____

_____

_____

_____

44. What causes gastric distention in patients receiving PPV and how can it be reduced?

_____

_____

_____

45. Why are medical and surgical patients subject to malnutrition during serious illness?

_____

_____

_____

46. List three deleterious effects that nutritional depletion can have on mechanically ventilated patients.

a. _____

b. _____

c. _____

47. What effects can overfeeding have on a mechanically ventilated patient?

_____

_____

_____

48. List five ways of assessing a patient's nutritional status.

    a. _____

    b. _____

    c. _____

    d. _____

    e. _____

49. How can some of the complications associated with mechanical ventilation be reduced?

    _____

    _____

    _____

CRITICAL THINKING QUESTIONS

1. Describe the cardiovascular effects, represented by the lettered arrows, that PPV is having on the heart in Figure 16-2.

    A. _____

    _____

    B. _____

    _____

    C. _____

    _____

    D. _____

    _____

CASE STUDIES

Case Study

A 30-year-old, 5-foot 8-inch, male postoperative patient with no lung disease is in the surgical intensive care unit receiving full mechanical support with the following ventilator settings: volume-controlled continuous mandatory ventilation (VC-CMV), rate 12 breaths/min, V_T 560 mL, flow rate 84 L/min, PEEP +10 cm H_2O, F_IO_2 0.5. His PIP is averaging around 30 cm H_2O and the plateau pressure is measured at 23 cm H_2O.

1. Calculate this patient's mean airway pressure.

   _____

   _____

   _____

   _____

   _____

2. Analyze the patient's arterial blood gas on these ventilator settings: pH 7.38, PCO_2 42 mm Hg, PO_2 78 mm Hg, S_aO_2 90%, HCO_3^- 23 mEq/L.

   _____

   _____

3. What is the most appropriate ventilator change at this time and why?

   _____

   _____

   _____

   _____

   _____

NBRC-STYLE QUESTIONS

1. What effect does the normal thoracic pump mechanism have on cardiac output (CO)?
   a. Reduces CO in normal individuals
   b. Improves CO in health individuals
   c. Improves CO in individuals with disease
   d. Improves CO in mechanically ventilated patients only

2. During PPV and PPV with PEEP, which of the following is true regarding the thoracic pump mechanism?
   a. CO is decreased and venous return is decreased.
   b. Left ventricular output is decreased and CO is increased.
   c. Left ventricular stroke volume is decreased and CO is decreased.
   d. Right heart venous return is increased and BP is increased.

3. The greatest reductions in venous return and cardiac output are most likely to occur during the use of which of the following ventilator modes?
   a. Continuous positive airway pressure (CPAP) 8 cm H_2O
   b. Intermittent mandatory volume (IMV) 10, V_T 450 mL
   c. CMV 12 with V_T 475 mL
   d. CMV 10, V_T 435 mL, PEEP +6 cm H_2O

4. A patient's inability to compensate for a diminished cardiac output during PPV will result in which of the following?
   a. Severe hemorrhaging
   b. Increased BP
   c. Compromised perfusion
   d. Maintenance of normal BP

5. For which of the following reasons are patients with acute respiratory distress syndrome are less likely to experience hemodynamic changes during PPV, even with high ventilatory pressures?
   a. They have elevated systemic BP.
   b. Their blood vessel walls have become too thick.
   c. Pressure is not transmitted to the pleural space.
   d. Pressure is lost in the poorly conductive airways.

6. Hazardous cardiovascular side effects in patients with severe bronchospasm are due to which of the following?
   a. Short inspiratory times
   b. Presence of auto-PEEP
   c. Elevated mean airway pressure
   d. Elevated peak inspiratory pressure

7. The pressure that has the most influence on the hemodynamic effects of PPV is which of the following?
   a. PEEP
   b. Peak pressure
   c. Plateau pressure
   d. Mean airway pressure

8. Methods of increasing mean airway pressure include which of the following?
   1. Increasing PEEP
   2. Increasing total cycle time
   3. Decreasing inspiratory time
   4. Adding an inflation hold
   a. 1 and 2 only
   b. 1 and 4 only
   c. 2 and 3 only
   d. 2 and 4 only

9. The risk of cardiovascular complications is least with the use of which of the following ventilator modes?
   a. Pressure-controlled (PC)-CMV
   b. VC-CMV with PEEP
   c. PC-IMV with pressure support
   d. CPAP with pressure support

10. The anticipated effects of PPV on the kidneys include which of the following?
    1. Diuresis
    2. Sodium retention
    3. Decreased urinary output
    4. Increased creatinine excretion
    a. 1 and 2 only
    b. 2 and 3 only
    c. 3 and 4 only
    d. 1 and 4 only

17 Effects of Positive-Pressure Ventilation on the Pulmonary System

LEARNING OBJECTIVES

On completion of this chapter, the reader will be able to do the following:

1. Recognize barotrauma or extra-alveolar air based on patient assessment.
2. Recommend appropriate action in patients with barotrauma.
3. Evaluate findings from a patient with acute respiratory distress syndrome to establish an optimum positive end-expiratory pressure (PEEP) and ventilation strategy.
4. Identify situations where chest wall rigidity can alter transpulmonary pressures and acceptable plateau pressures.
5. Name the types of ventilator-induced lung injury (VILI) caused by opening and closing of alveoli and overdistention of alveoli.
6. Compare the clinical findings in hyperventilation and hypoventilation.
7. Recommend ventilator settings in patients with hyperventilation and hypoventilation.
8. Identify a patient with air trapping.
9. Provide strategies to reduce auto-PEEP.
10. Suggest methods to reduce the work of breathing (WOB) during mechanical ventilation.
11. List the possible responses to an increase in mean airway pressure in a ventilated patient.
12. Describe the effects of positive-pressure ventilation (PPV) on pulmonary gas distribution and pulmonary perfusion in relation to normal spontaneous breathing.

159

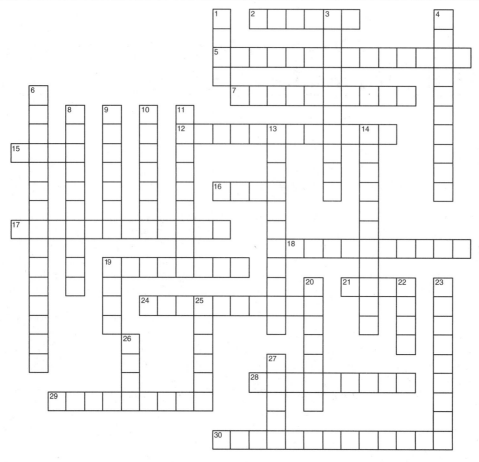

Across

2 Like blebs, these focal regions in the chest wall increases risk of rupture of the lung
5 Caused by too much volume in the alveoli
7 Occurs with overdistention of more compliant areas of the lung
12 General name for mediators released as a result of lung injury
15 Type of asynchrony caused by more than one breathe type delivered by the ventilator
16 Abbreviation for lung injury at the level of the acinus
17 Described as alveolar rupture, interstitial emphysema, or perivascular and alveolar hemorrhage, which can eventually lead to death
18 Circulation of mediators cause this type of failure
19 Maneuver that causes pleural pressure to be positive
21 Asynchrony caused by inappropriate baseline settings
24 Type of trauma caused by high levels of pressure
28 One type of mediator released as a result of lung injury
29 Touching subcutaneous emphysema feels like this
30 Closing of lung units

Down

1 Asynchrony caused by inadequate gas speed
3 Atelectasis caused by high oxygen concentration
4 Asynchrony caused by dual control modes of ventilation (two words)
6 Inadequate alveolar ventilation
8 The sign indicative of a tension pneumothorax on chest radiograph (two words)
9 Type of hyperinflation caused by failure of lung volume to return to passive functional residual capacity
10 Asynchrony caused by inappropriate sensitivity settings
11 Caused by release of inflammatory mediators from the lungs
13 A pneumothorax causes this to shift
14 Opening of lung units
19 Abbreviation for lung injury as a consequence of mechanical ventilation
20 Asynchrony may cause this type of chest-abdominal movement
22 Vascular area that hemorrhages due to alveolar trauma
23 This area of the lungs receives most blood flow in the supine position
25 Another name for auto-PEEP or intrinsic PEEP
26 Abbreviation for diaphragm's electrical activity
27 Asynchrony caused by a very long inspiratory time

CHAPTER REVIEW QUESTIONS

1. Define *volutrauma*, *biotrauma*, and *atelectrauma*.

2. Briefly describe the difference between VILI and ventilator-associated lung injury.

3. List five conditions that can predispose a patient to barotrauma while he or she is being mechanically ventilated.

   a.
   b.
   c.
   d.
   e.

4. During patient ventilator system checks the respiratory therapist notes the right lateral side of the patient's neck and face appear puffy. These areas feel crepitant to the touch; however, no distress is observed in the patient. What is the most likely cause of this problem?

5. What is likely the cause of a sudden onset of increased peak airway pressures and hyper-resonance in a patient receiving mechanical ventilation?

6. What is the treatment for a tension pneumothorax?

7. When a mechanically ventilated patient develops a tension pneumothorax, how should they be ventilated until the appropriate treatment can begin?

8. List four clinical signs of a tension pneumothorax.

   a.
   b.
   c.
   d.

9. How would a chest radiograph of a patient with a tension pneumothorax look?

10. Air dissecting into the retroperitoneal space is known as _____ .

11. What is the minimum transpulmonary pressure that has been associated with lung injury in animals?

12. List three examples of clinical situations where lung injury can occur from high transpulmonary pressure.

   a.
   b.
   c.

13. Describe how volutrauma occurs.

14. What are the three primary types of lung injury that can occur with the repeated opening and closing of lung units? Briefly explain each.

   a.
   b.
   c.

15. Explain shear stress and how it can lead to edema formation.

16. Define atelectrauma and give a clinical situation puts a ventilated patient at risk of developing it.

_____

_____

17. List two chemical mediators that are released when the alveolar epithelial cells are overstretched.

a. _____

b. _____

18. Describe how multiorgan dysfunction syndrome develops in a patient receiving mechanical ventilation.

_____

_____

_____

_____

19. How can multiorgan dysfunction syndrome be avoided during mechanical ventilation?

_____

_____

_____

20. In what areas of the lung are ventilation and perfusion best matched during spontaneous ventilation in the supine position?

_____

_____

21. Describe how ventilation and perfusion are altered during PPV in a patient who is sedated and paralyzed.

_____

_____

_____

_____

22. How can the changes in gas distribution during mechanical ventilation be minimized?

_____

23. How can PPV increase dead space?

_____

_____

_____

24. Why would the use of high volumes during PPV and PEEP cause an increase in pulmonary shunting?

_____

_____

_____

_____

25. How can mechanical ventilation cause an increase in pulmonary vascular resistance?

_____

_____

_____

26. Explain how hypoventilation can lead to cardiac dysrhythmias.

_____

27. What type of patient may benefit from permissive hypercapnia?

_____

28. List four reasons for patient-induced hyperventilation.

a. _____

b. _____

c. _____

d. _____

29. What acid-base disturbance can cause a right shift in the oxygen dissociation curve?

_____

30. Describe two clinical implications of prolonged ventilator-induced hyperventilation?

a. _____

_____

b. _____

_____

31. What happens to the cerebrospinal fluid during prolonged hyperventilation during mechanical ventilation?

_____

_____

_____

_____

32. When is the administration of intravenous bicarbonate indicated?

_____

_____

33. List four causes of metabolic alkalosis in the clinical setting.

a. _____

b. _____

c. _____

d. _____

34. What can cause auto-PEEP without dynamic hyperinflation?

_____

_____

35. Describe how ventilator-induced auto-PEEP can be created.

_____

_____

_____

_____

_____

36. What patient factors increase the risk of auto-PEEP?

_____

_____

_____

37. On the graph below, draw a flow-time curve for volume-controlled continuous mandatory ventilation (VC-CMV), showing a "normal" exhalation and one exhibiting auto-PEEP.

_____

_____

38. What technique is used to detect the presence of auto-PEEP?

_____

39. How many time constants are necessary for the lungs to empty 98% of the inspired volume?

_____

40. Define dynamic hyperinflation.

_____

_____

41. What effects can the presence of auto-PEEP have on ventilator function?

_____

_____

_____

_____

_____

Chapter **17** **Effects of Positive-Pressure Ventilation on the Pulmonary System**

42. Calculate static compliance for the following situation: V_T 525 mL, peak inspiratory pressure (PIP) 43 cm H_2O, $P_{plateau}$ 30 cm H_2O, set PEEP 12 cm H_2O, auto-PEEP 5 cm H_2O.

_____

_____

_____

_____

43. List four strategies that can be used to decrease auto-PEEP when the patient is receiving full ventilatory support.

a. _____

b. _____

c. _____

d. _____

44. List four modes of ventilation that may be used to decrease auto-PEEP in a patient who is intubated and has spontaneous breathing efforts.

a. _____

b. _____

c. _____

d. _____

45. When does pulmonary oxygen toxicity become a problem in adults and premature infants?

_____

_____

_____

46. If an F_IO_2 of greater than _____ is required, PEEP should be used. List four ways to assess pulmonary changes associated with oxygen toxicity.

a. _____

b. _____

c. _____

d. _____

47. What are the lower limit targets for oxygenation for patients receiving mechanical ventilation?

_____

48. The use of low tidal volumes with oxygen concentrations greater than 70% may lead to

_____.

49. What is the normal inspiratory WOB?

_____

50. When is inspiratory WOB considered high?

_____

51. What are some signs a patient has an increased WOB?

_____

52. Calculate the estimated WOB for a patient receiving mechanical ventilation with the following data: PIP = 45 cm H_2O, $P_{plateau}$ = 33 cm H_2O, and V_T = 475 mL.

_____

_____

_____

_____

53. List four basic strategies for minimizing a patient's WOB.

a. _____

b. _____

c. _____

d. _____

54. List four signs of patient-ventilator dyssynchrony.

a. _____

b. _____

c. _____

d. _____

55. Define trigger asynchrony and describe a method to avoid it.

_____

_____

_____

56. How can auto-PEEP cause trigger asynchrony?

_____

_____

_____

57. What should the initial flow be set at when using volume ventilation with a constant flow?

_____

58. What type of breaths may provide more synchrony for a patient with high flow demands and why?

_____

_____

_____

59. What adjustment can be made during pressure-targeted ventilation to lessen the rapid rise of flow when a breath begins?

_____

_____

60. What is cycle dyssynchrony and under what conditions can it occur?

_____

_____

_____

61. What strategies may be used to eliminate cycle dyssynchrony during mechanical ventilation with full support and spontaneous ventilation?

_____

_____

_____

62. What mode of ventilation delivers varying breath types, which may result in mode dyssynchrony?

_____

63. When does PEEP asynchrony occur?

_____

_____

64. How can closed-loop ventilation lead to asynchrony?

_____

_____

_____

_____

65. List five potential mechanical failures that can occur during mechanical ventilation.

a. _____

b. _____

c. _____

d. _____

e. _____

66. List seven potential mechanical failures that can occur with mechanical ventilation.

a. _____

b. _____

c. _____

d. _____

e. _____

f. _____

g. _____

67. What hazards are associated with the use of both heat moisture exchangers and heated humidifiers?

_____

_____

_____

Questions 1 and 2 refer to the figure below.

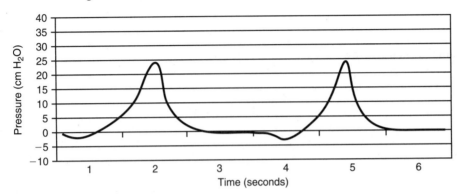

1. What problem is shown in this pressure-time curve?

_____

2. What change can be made to the ventilator settings to alleviate this problem?

_____

Questions 3 and 4 refer to the figure below.

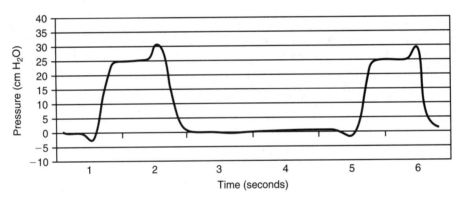

3. What problem is shown in this pressure-time curve?

_____

4. What change can be made to the ventilator settings to alleviate this problem?

_____

5. Which of the following patients will be more likely to develop auto-PEEP due to dynamic hyperinflation with a set rate of 12 breaths/min? Why?

Patient #1: airway resistance = 25 cm H_2O/L/s and static compliance = 50 mL/cm H_2O

Patient #2: airway resistance = 6 cm H_2O/L/s and static compliance = 25 mL/cm H_2O

_____

_____

_____

_____

Case Study 1

A patient 4 days post single-lung transplant is being mechanically ventilated. The remaining lung is fibrotic on chest radiograph and the transplanted lung is hyperinflated. The patient is unresponsive, cyanotic, and hypotensive. Her ideal body weight is 135 pounds. She is being ventilated with VC-CMV and the flow sheet for the past few hours shows the following:

Time	Set Rate	Set V_T	Flow	PIP	F_iO_2	PEEP	pH	PCO_2	PO_2
0800	20	300	60	52	0.7	0	7.18	86	275
1000	22	300	60	50	1.0	0	7.15	94	504
1200	24	300	60	55	1.0	0	7.14	95	95
1400	40	320	60	60	1.0	0	7.06	110	125

$P_{plateau}$ at 1400 hours was 38 cm H_2O.

1. What is the most apparent problem in this patient's ventilator course?

2. What is the most likely cause of this problem?

3. What complications is this patient at risk of developing?

4. What should be the first change made to this patient's ventilator parameters?

Case Study 2

A 65-year-old, 5-foot 10-inch, male patient with chronic obstructive pulmonary disease (COPD) was intubated 3 days ago and is being mechanically ventilated with VC-CMV rate 14 breaths/min, V_T 550 mL, F_iO_2 0.3, and PEEP +3 cm H_2O. This patient's baseline room air arterial blood gas (ABG) is pH 7.37, P_aCO_2 57 mm Hg, P_aO_2 54 mm Hg, S_aO_2 90%, and HCO_3^- 30 mEq/L. The ABGs on the current ventilator setting are pH 7.41, $PaCO_2$ 41 mm Hg, P_aO_2 70 mm Hg, S_aO_2 94%, and HCO_3^- 25 mEq/L. The patient is placed on volume-controlled intermittent mandatory ventilation (VC-IMV) to begin the weaning process and the mandatory rate is reduced to 6 breaths/min.

One hour after this change the respiratory therapist is called to the patient's room because the high respiratory rate alarm is sounding. The patient is diaphoretic, anxious, tachycardic, and is using accessory muscles.

1. What is the most likely cause of this patient's failure to wean?

2. What could the respiratory therapist do to alleviate this problem?

_____

_____

_____

_____

3. After 48 hours, the volume-controlled synchronized intermittent mandatory ventilation (VC-SIMV) is switched to pressure-support ventilation 10 cm H_2O. The respiratory therapist observes the pressure-time scalar shown below. What is causing the spike at the end of the wave?

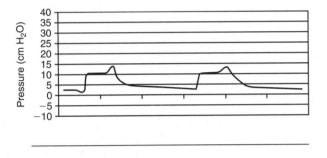

_____

_____

4. How can the problem be alleviated?

_____

Case Study 3

A 33 year-old male was endotracheal intubated for 3 hours for a surgical procedure. He was extubated after 1 day of mechanical ventilation. Thirty minutes after extubation, the nurse calls you and states he is experiencing shortness of breath. When you enter his room you can hear stridor.

1. What is stridor?

2. What is the likely cause of stridor in this patient?

3. How would you begin assessment on this patient?

4. How would you treat him to alleviate the problem?

1. The major hazard(s) of oxygen therapy in association with mechanical ventilation include which of the following?
   1. Tachycardia
   2. Absorption atelectasis
   3. Oxygen-induced bradypnea
   4. Pulmonary oxygen toxicity
   a. 3 only
   b. 1 and 2 only
   c. 2 and 4 only
   d. 1, 3, and 4 only

2. Auto-PEEP should be suspected during which of the following observations?
   a. There is a prolonged postexpiratory pause.
   b. The patient coughs severely when suctioned.
   c. Expiration is continuous up to the next inspiration.
   d. The SIMV mandatory rate is set at 10 breaths/min.

3. The lung capacity that increases when auto-PEEP is present is which of the following?
   a. Vital capacity
   b. Inspiratory capacity
   c. Total lung capacity
   d. Functional residual capacity

4. Iatrogenic hyperventilation of a patient with a diagnosis of COPD may lead to which of the following consequences?
   1. Tetany
   2. Air trapping
   3. Cerebral edema
   4. Hypokalemia
   a. 2 only
   b. 1 and 3 only
   c. 2 and 4 only
   d. 1, 2, and 4 only

5. A patient who has been mechanically ventilated for 7 days has recently developed subcutaneous emphysema. Further assessment reveals cyanosis, signs of dyspnea, and a markedly elevated PIP. This patient is most likely experiencing which of the following?
   a. Pneumothorax
   b. Pneumoperitoneum
   c. Increased compliance
   d. Pneumomediastinum

6. The risk of volutrauma is increased for mechanically ventilated patients who exhibit which of the following?
   a. Increased PTA
   b. Decreased PA
   c. Increased PL
   d. Decreased P_{AO}

7. The amount of bicarbonate replacement given to a patient with severe metabolic acidosis who weighs 145 pounds and has a base deficit of 10 should be which of the following?
   a. 55 mEq
   b. 110 mEq
   c. 220 mEq
   d. 242 mEq

8. Failure to recognize a patient's trigger efforts is known as which of the following?
   a. Mode dyssynchrony
   b. Flow dyssynchrony
   c. Trigger dyssynchrony
   d. Closed-loop ventilation dyssynchrony

9. An increase in a patient's assist rate followed by a rise in PIP and drop in exhaled tidal volume is most often associated with which of the following?
   a. Auto-PEEP
   b. Mode dyssynchrony
   c. PEEP dyssynchrony
   d. Subcutaneous emphysema

10. The presence of fine, late inspiratory crackles may reflect which of the following lung injuries?
    1. Biotrauma
    2. Shear stress
    3. Surfactant alteration
    4. Subcutaneous emphysema
   a. 1 and 2 only
   b. 2 and 3 only
   c. 1 and 4 only
   d. 3 and 4 only

18 Problem Solving and Troubleshooting

On completion of this chapter, the reader will be able to do the following:

1. Identify various types of technical problems encountered during mechanical ventilation of critically ill patients and describe the steps that can be used to protect a patient when problems occur.
2. Name at least two possible causes for each of the following alarm situations: low-pressure alarm, high-pressure alarm, low positive end-expiratory pressure (PEEP)/continuous positive airway pressure (CPAP) alarms, apnea alarm, low or high tidal volume alarm, low or high minute volume alarm, low or high respiratory rate alarm, low or high F_IO_2 alarm, low source gas pressure or power input alarm, ventilator inoperative alarm, and technical error message.
3. Determine the cause of a problem using a graphic from a patient-ventilator system.
4. Assess a description of a patient situation and recommend a solution.
5. Describe the signs and symptoms associated with patient-ventilator asynchrony.
6. Explain the correct procedure for determining whether a problem originates with the patient or with the ventilator in patient-ventilator asynchrony.
7. List four ways the addition of a nebulizer powered by an external source gas can affect ventilator function.
8. Recognize abnormalities in ventilator graphics and patient response in the event of inadequate gas flow delivery to a patient.
9. Identify potential problems related to electrolyte imbalances and their causes.
10. Recognize the signs and symptoms of a respiratory infection.
11. Identify a problem associated with an artificial airway or a mask used for noninvasive positive-pressure ventilation.
12. Recognize the presence of auto-PEEP using ventilator graphics.
13. Suggest appropriate interventions for a patient who has experienced a right mainstem intubation and for a patient with a pneumothorax, using physical assessment data.
14. Describe potential problems associated with using a heated humidification system during mechanical ventilation.
15. Use a ventilator flow-volume loop to assess a patient's response to bronchodilator therapy.
16. Make recommendations about ventilator parameters for a patient with acute respiratory distress syndrome.
17. Recommend adjustment of flow-cycle criteria during pressure support ventilation based on ventilator graphics.

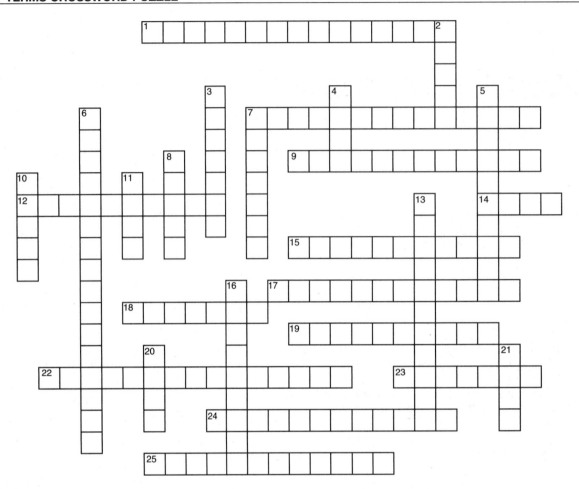

Across

1 The type of interference caused by a cell phone
7 Fluid in the lungs (two words)
9 A life-threatening cause of severe patient distress seen in patients receiving positive-pressure ventilation
12 The artery whose wall may be eroded and can rupture within 3 weeks after a tracheostomy
14 Continuous suction endotracheal tube (abbreviation)
15 An indicator of cardiopulmonary distress
18 Waveform _____ is caused by oscillation of air in the patient-ventilator circuit at the beginning of inspiration
19 Without synchrony
22 Identification and resolution of technical malfunctions in the patient-ventilator system
23 Abnormal accumulation of edematous fluid within the peritoneal cavity
24 Smooth muscle contraction in the lungs
25 A type of therapy that breaks up blood clots

Down

2 Active exhalation during pressure-support ventilation is a common cause of this type of dyssynchrony
3 A situation in which one finds discord or in which one is uncomfortable and does not have an immediate solution
4 This type of dyssynchrony occurs when more than one breath type is delivered
5 Inward protrusion of intercostal spaces
6 Blood clot in the lungs (two words)
7 The person attached to the ventilator
8 An alert for a clinician, it can be visual or audible
10 The bronchus that an endotracheal tube can most easily slip into
11 An unintentional bend in the endotracheal tube
13 Especially profuse perspiration
16 Radiograph of blood vessels
20 The type of dyssynchrony that occurs when gas speed is inadequate
21 A hole in a endotracheal tube cuff may cause this

CHAPTER REVIEW QUESTIONS

1. Define the term *problem*.

2. Define *troubleshooting* in the context of mechanical ventilation.

3. When responding to an activated ventilator alarm, what is the respiratory therapist's first priority?

4. What assessments must be made following response to an activated ventilator alarm?

5. If a serious ventilatory problem is detected, what should the respiratory therapist do?

6. List the advantages and disadvantages of manually ventilating a patient when a problem with the ventilator is detected.

7. List five physical signs of distress that a patient receiving mechanical ventilation might exhibit.

   a.
   b.
   c.
   d.
   e.

8. What equipment, techniques, or data can be used to help identify the cause of a patient's sudden distress while being mechanically ventilated?

9. List six patient-related causes of sudden respiratory distress that originate within the patient's lungs.

   a.
   b.
   c.
   d.
   e.
   f.

10. List six nonpulmonary patient-related causes of sudden respiratory distress.

    a.
    b.
    c.
    d.
    e.
    f.

11. Aside from patient-ventilator asynchrony, what ventilator-related issues can cause sudden respiratory distress in patients?

12. How should the respiratory therapist distinguish the difference between severe distress caused by a ventilator-related or patient-related problem?

13. Describe the seven steps needed to manage sudden severe distress in a ventilator-supported patient.

    a. _____

    b. _____

    c. _____

    d. _____

    e. _____

    f. _____

    g. _____

14. An oral endotracheal tube should be approximately at what mark for men and for women? What are the appropriate ranges for each?

    _____

    _____

15. What steps should be taken if a suction catheter cannot be passed down the endotracheal tube of a patient in severe respiratory distress (patient is not biting the tube)?

    _____

    _____

16. What clinical manifestation should a respiratory therapist look for when a tension pneumothorax is suspected during positive-pressure ventilation?

    _____

    _____

    _____

17. If a tension pneumothorax is strongly suspected and cardiopulmonary arrest is imminent, what action should be taken?

    _____

    _____

18. What signs suggest that a patient is experiencing bronchospasm while receiving mechanical ventilation?

    _____

    _____

    _____

19. How can problems due to secretions be minimized during mechanical ventilation?

    _____

    _____

    _____

20. What is the difference in onset between cardiogenic and noncardiogenic pulmonary edema?

    _____

    _____

    _____

21. How does auto-PEEP affect the flow-time scalar and the flow-volume loop?

    _____

    _____

22. List three conditions that may stimulate the respiratory center output.

    a. _____

    b. _____

    c. _____

23. Describe how the presence of abdominal distention can cause atelectasis, ventilation/perfusion abnormalities, and hypoxemia?

    _____

    _____

    _____

24. The rapid onset of hypoxemia, tachycardia, tachypnea, and hypertension, along with a decrease in end-tidal CO_2, is indicative of what type of patient problem? How can this problem be confirmed and treated?

    _____

    _____

    _____

25. List four sources of leaks in the patient-ventilator system to occur.

    a. _____

    b. _____

    c. _____

    d. _____

26. List four common causes of a low-pressure alarm situation.

a. _____

b. _____

c. _____

d. _____

27. List nine common causes of a high-pressure alarm situation.

a. _____

b. _____

c. _____

d. _____

e. _____

f. _____

g. _____

h. _____

i. _____

28. If the peak inspiratory pressure (PIP) is 30 cm H_2O, what should the low- and high-pressure alarms be set at?

_____

_____

29. Name two conditions that would trigger a low PEEP/CPAP alarm.

a. _____

b. _____

30. List five potential causes for triggering an apnea alarm.

a. _____

b. _____

c. _____

d. _____

e. _____

31. List two potential causes for triggering a low-source gas pressure alarm.

a. _____

b. _____

32. List two potential causes for a power-input alarm.

a. _____

b. _____

33. What is the most likely cause of a "ventilator inoperative" alarm?

_____

_____

34. Describe the alarm situations and ventilator graphics that a leak in the patient-ventilator system would cause.

_____

_____

_____

_____

35. What types of graphics will allow the respiratory therapist to detect inadequate flow?

_____

_____

_____

36. The phenomenon caused by the oscillation of air in the patient-ventilator circuit and at the upper airway at the beginning of inspiration is known as

_____

37. What can be done to alleviate the problem caused by the phenomenon in Question 36?

_____

_____

38. List three problems that may cause the expiratory portion of the volume-time curve to go below baseline.

a. _____

b. _____

c. _____

39. How does an externally powered nebulizer affect ventilator function?

_____

_____

_____

_____

40. A leak in the endotracheal tube cuff will cause which alarms to be activated?

_____

_____

41. Compare the findings from a right mainstem intubation and from a left and right tension pneumothorax by completing the chart below.

Clinical Findings	Right Mainstem Intubation	Left-sided Pneumothorax	Right-sided Pneumothorax
PIP	_____	_____	_____
$P_{plateau}$	_____	_____	_____
Breath sounds	_____	_____	_____
Chest movement	_____	_____	_____
Percussion	_____	_____	_____
Tracheal shift	_____	_____	_____

42. During mechanical ventilation with pressure controlled-continuous mandatory ventilation (PC-CMV), the low tidal volume alarm becomes activated on every breath; there is no leak in the system. What could be the cause of this alarm?

_____

_____

43. What situations can cause the inspiratory-to-expiratory ratio indicator and alarm to be activated?

_____

_____

_____

44. A respiratory therapist responding to a ventilator alarm finds that the high respiratory rate alarm is activated. The ventilator is set to volume-controlled-continuous mandatory ventilation (VC-CMV) rate 12. What are some possible reasons for this activated alarm?

_____

_____

_____

CRITICAL THINKING QUESTIONS

Questions 1 through 4 refer to the following scenario.

You are the respiratory therapist who responds to a sounding ventilator alarm. The patient has been receiving mechanical ventilation for the past 3 days following an exacerbation of congestive heart failure and pneumonia. She has been unresponsive to verbal stimuli during this period. Her ventilator settings are VC-CMV, set rate 12 breaths/min, tidal volume 475 mL, F_IO_2 0.5, and PEEP +5 cm H_2O. The PIP has been averaging 28 cm H_2O, and the $P_{plateau}$ about 21 cm H_2O. As you approach the patient you note that the alarm panel indicates a high-pressure condition along with low exhaled tidal volume and low exhaled minute volume. The patient's high-pressure alarm threshold is set at 40 cm H_2O and the returned volume is 175 mL.

1. What action should the respiratory therapist take at this time?

_____

_____

_____

2. Name three conditions that could cause this situation.

a. _____

b. _____

c. _____

3. Describe the best course of action to remedy each of the three conditions mentioned in the previous answer.

_____

_____

_____

_____

4. Why are the low exhaled tidal volume and low exhaled minute volume active along with the high-pressure alarm?

_____

_____

_____

_____

_____

Questions 5 and 6 refer to the following scenario.

A patient recently weaned from full ventilatory support has just been switched to CPAP $+10$ cm H_2O with pressure support of 25 cm H_2O. After a few spontaneous breaths on the CPAP with pressure support, the patient developed respiratory distress. The patient does not seem to be able to trigger the pressure-supported breaths and the ventilator's apnea alarm has been activated.

5. Explain two possible causes for this patient's respiratory distress.

a. _____

b. _____

6. What actions could correct these possible causes?

_____

_____

_____

CASE STUDIES

Case Study 1

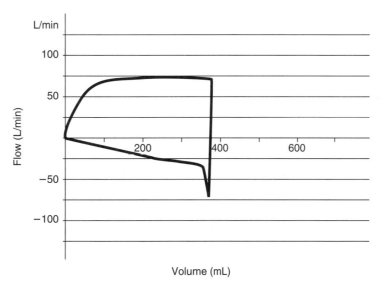

1. The flow-volume loop shown in the Figure 18-1 is for a patient receiving mechanical ventilation. What type of problem is demonstrated in this flow-volume loop?

_____

2. What can be done to solve this problem?

_____

Case Study 2

A 42-year-old male had surgery to repair a crushed hip and femur fractures that occurred in a motor vehicle crash. Five hours after surgery, the patient continues to receive positive-pressure ventilation. Till now the patient's condition has been stable, but he has been unconscious. At 1810 hours, a sudden change in the patient's vital signs has brought the respiratory therapist to the patient's bedside. The pulse oximetry reading has dropped from 96 to 87%, and blood pressure (BP) has risen from 136/82 to 160/100 mm Hg. The table below shows the last patient-ventilator checks.

Date	5/29	5/29	5/29	5/29
Time	1400	1610	1750	1810
Mode	PC-CMV	PC-CMV	PC-CMV	PC-CMV
Set rate	12	12	12	12
Total rate	12	12	20	25
Volume with set PIP	620 mL	628 mL	625 mL	615 mL
T_I	1 second	1 second	1 second	1 second
Waveform	Square	Square	Square	Square
PIP (cm H_2O)	30	28	32	33
$P_{plateau}$ (cm H_2O)	23	21	22	20
PEEP (cm H_2O)	5	5	5	↑ 8
F_IO_2	0.4	0.4	0.4	↑ 0.6
Breath sounds	Bilateral clear	Bilateral clear	Bilateral clear	Bilateral clear
BP (mm Hg)	136/82	132/80	155/88	160/100
Heart rate (BPM)	96	94	125	128
SpO_2	96%	96%	96%	87%
$P_{ET}CO_2$ (mm Hg)	36	36	34	26
Arterial blood gases				
pH	7.43	—	—	7.47
$PaCO_2$ (mm Hg)	39	—	—	30
P_aO_2 (mm Hg)	98	—	—	78

1. The patient is now in obvious respiratory distress. What action should the respiratory therapist take at this time?

_____

_____

2. Nothing that is done seems to relieve this patient's respiratory distress. What is the most likely cause of this problem?

_____

_____

Case Study 3

A 62-year-old woman is receiving ventilatory support with volume ventilation. She had abdominal surgery 10 hours ago. She has no history of smoking. Over the past few hours, the following patient information was gathered.

Time	0700	0900	1000
Volume	450 mL	450 mL	450 mL
PIP	18 cm H_2O	24 cm H_2O	27 cm H_2O
$P_{plateau}$	13 cm H_2O	12 cm H_2O	14 cm H_2O

1. What is the most likely cause of the increase in PIP between 7 and 10 AM?

_____

_____

2. List some of the problems that can cause this type of increase in PIP.

_____

_____

3. What actions should the respiratory therapist take to determine the source of this patient's problem?

_____

_____

NBRC-STYLE QUESTIONS

1. During pressure-control ventilation, the alarm that identifies worsening lung compliance is which of the following?
   a. Low PEEP/CPAP
   b. High respiratory rate
   c. Low V_T
   d. High PIP

2. Identify the problem in the following flow-time scalar.

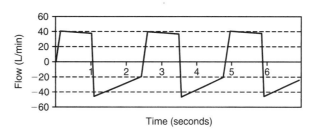

   a. Auto-PEEP
   b. Excessively prolonged T_E
   c. Inadequate T_I
   d. Increased airway resistance

3. Which of the following may solve the problem represented in the pressure-time scalar in below?

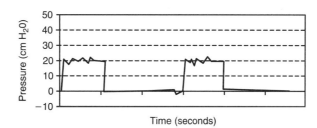

   a. Changing the flow waveform
   b. Increasing pressure sensitivity
   c. Increasing inspiratory rise time
   d. Increasing the peak pressure

Chapter **18** **Problem Solving and Troubleshooting**

4. The problem indicated in the flow-volume loop below is which of the following?

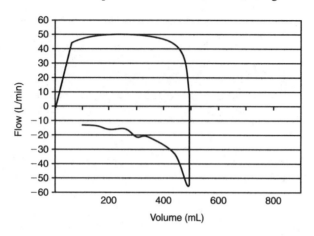

a. Increase in airway resistance
b. Active exhalation against inspiration
c. Leak in the patient-ventilator system
d. Auto-PEEP

5. The problem indicated in the pressure-volume loop below, obtained during VC-CMV, can be solved by which of the following?

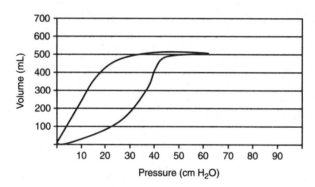

1. Suctioning of the endotracheal tube
2. Switching to PC-CMV
3. Lower the V_T in VC-CMV
4. Administering a bronchodilator
a. 1 and 2
b. 2 and 3
c. 3 and 4
d. 1 and 4

6. The problem that could cause the pressure-time scalar below is which of the following?

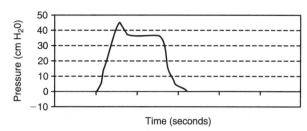

Time (seconds)

1. Bronchoconstriction
2. High airway resistance
3. Alveolar overdistention
4. Decreased lung compliance
   a. 1 and 2
   b. 2 and 3
   c. 3 and 4
   d. 1 and 4

7. The respiratory therapist is assessing a mechanically ventilated patient who has developed sudden respiratory distress. The respiratory therapist notes that the 15-mm endotracheal tube adapter is at the level of the patient's teeth. The suspected airway problem is which of the following?
   a. Cuff rupture or leakage
   b. Rupture of the innominate artery
   c. Patient biting the endotracheal tube
   d. The endotracheal tube has slipped into the right mainstem bronchus

8. The respiratory therapist is unable to pass a suction catheter into a patient's endotracheal tube or to ventilate the patient manually with a resuscitator bag. Deflation of the cuff does not relieve the patient's distress. The most appropriate action is which of the following?
   a. Reinflate the cuff and attempt ventilation again.
   b. Remove the endotracheal tube and provide bag-mask ventilation.
   c. Keep the cuff inflated and attempt ventilation again with 100% oxygen.
   d. Deflate the cuff, suction the upper airway, and provide bag-mask ventilation.

9. The respiratory therapist strongly suspects that the patient has a tension pneumothorax. What treatment would the respiratory therapist assist the physician with to alleviate this life-threatening situation?
   a. Suction the patient's endotracheal tube vigorously
   b. Insert a chest tube into the sixth intercostal space
   c. Insert a 14- or 16-gauge needle into the second intercostal space
   d. Remove the patient from the ventilator and provide resuscitation

10. While providing mechanical ventilatory support for a conscious patient, the respiratory therapist notes dyspnea, wheezing, and increased use of accessory muscles of breathing. These clinical findings are most closely associated with which of the following?
    a. Cuff leakage
    b. Bronchospasm
    c. Pneumothorax
    d. Increased secretions

Chapter **18** **Problem Solving and Troubleshooting**

11. What should the respiratory therapist check first when a low-pressure alarm is activated on a ventilator?
    a. Apnea parameters
    b. Patient connection
    c. 50 psi gas source
    d. Ventilator electronics

12. What problem must be present to cause simultaneous activation of the low-pressure, low-volume, and low minute ventilation alarms?
    a. Inadequate flow setting
    b. Ventilator dyssynchrony
    c. Patient-ventilator system leak
    d. Inappropriate trigger sensitivity

19 Basic Concepts of Noninvasive Positive-Pressure Ventilation

LEARNING OBJECTIVES

Upon completion of this chapter, the reader will be able to do the following:

1. Define *noninvasive ventilation* and discuss the three basic noninvasive techniques.
2. Discuss the clinical and physiologic benefits of noninvasive positive-pressure ventilation (NIV).
3. Identify the selection and exclusion criteria for NIV application in the acute and chronic care settings.
4. Compare the types of ventilators used for noninvasive ventilation.
5. Explain the importance of humidification during NIV application.
6. Describe the factors that will influence the F_IO_2 from a portable pressure-targeted ventilator.
7. Identify possible causes of rebreathing CO_2 during NIV administration from a portable pressure-targeted ventilator.
8. Compare the advantages and disadvantages of the various types of interfaces for the application of NIV.
9. List the steps used in the initiation of NIV.
10. Discuss several factors that affect the delivery of aerosols during NIV.
11. Identify several indicators of success for patients on NIV.
12. Make recommendations for ventilator changes based on observation of the patient's respiratory status, acid-base status, or oxygenation status.
13. Recognize potential complications of NIV.
14. Provide optional solutions to complications of NIV.
15. Describe two basic approaches to weaning a patient from NIV.

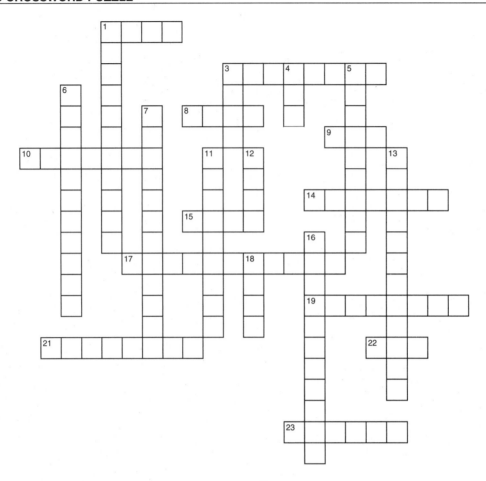

Across

1 First-choice therapy for the treatment of obstructive sleep apnea (OSA)
3 Type of ventilator used during the polio epidemic (two words)
8 A therapy used to deliver aerosolized medication periodically with positive pressure breaths (abbreviation)
9 Another name for bilevel continuous positive airway pressure (CPAP) ventilators (abbreviation)
10 A symptom of chronic hypoventilation
14 A type of sleep apnea that originates in the brain
15 A setting that allows positive pressure levels to gradually increase
17 Medication given to treat gastric insufflation
19 A type of heated humidifier the has been shown to reduce drying of the nasal mucosa during NIV
21 A type of mask that covers both nose and mouth
22 Abbreviation for a type of pneumonia acquired outside the hospital
23 The material that fastens the head gear

Down

1 A type of pulmonary edema due to a weak heart
3 Uses a pressure-targeted ventilator and a mask (abbreviation)
4 Noninvasive positive-pressure ventilation (abbreviation)
5 A type of hypoventilation that occurs at night
6 Type of sleep apnea that occurs from the collapse of the upper airway during sleep
7 A portable negative pressure device (two words)
11 The setting that controls the amount of time it takes for the positive pressure level to gradually increase (two words)
12 The expiratory setting for bilevel CPAP (abbreviation)
13 Right-sided heart failure due to an obstructive pulmonary disease (two words)
16 Secretions that are dried up are _____
18 The inspiratory setting for bilevel CPAP (abbreviation)

CHAPTER REVIEW QUESTIONS

1. Define *NIV*.

   _____

   _____

2. What are the three basic methods of applying NIV?

   a. _____

   b. _____

   c. _____

3. Explain how negative-pressure ventilators (body ventilators) work.

   _____

   _____

   _____

   _____

   _____

   _____

4. Name two negative-pressure ventilators.

   a. _____

   b. _____

5. What is the most significant benefit of NIV?

   _____

6. What is the primary goal of NIV in the acute care setting?

   _____

7. List six clinical benefits of NIV in the acute care setting.

   a. _____

   b. _____

   c. _____

   d. _____

   e. _____

   f. _____

8. List three clinical benefits of NIV in the chronic care setting.

   a. _____

   b. _____

   c. _____

9. Describe how the use of NIV in acute respiratory failure improve gas exchange.

   _____

   _____

10. Explain the benefits of using NIV via a facemask instead of invasive mechanical ventilation in the treatment of acute respiratory failure due to chronic obstructive pulmonary disease (COPD).

    _____

    _____

    _____

11. What benefit was seen when using NIV for COPD patients with community-acquired pneumonia (CAP)?

    _____

    _____

    _____

12. When a patient with cardiogenic pulmonary edema does not respond to conventional pharmacologic and oxygen therapy, what types of NIV have been shown to be effective?

    _____

    _____

    _____

13. List four clinical disorders that manifest in chronic respiratory failure which require NIV as supportive therapy.

    a. _____

    b. _____

    c. _____

    d. _____

14. List five symptoms of chronic hypoventilation.

    a. _____

    b. _____

    c. _____

    d. _____

    e. _____

15. Approximately how many hours must a patient with chronic hypoventilation use NIV to achieve clinical benefits?

    _____

16. Describe the clinical benefits of using NIV only at night or intermittently during the day for patients with neuromuscular disorders.

    _____

    _____

    _____

17. List the criteria for using NIV with patients who have chronic stable COPD.

    _____

    _____

    _____

18. Jane is a 22-year-old patient with advanced cystic fibrosis. She asks you if NIV could benefit her. How would you respond?

    _____

    _____

19. What may be the next course of treatment for an OSA patient that continues to hypoventilate and experience nocturnal desaturation while receiving CPAP?

    _____

    _____

20. Mrs. T is concerned you are attempting to remove her husband from invasive ventilation too soon. She is worried he may become short of breath again despite the physician's assurance he is ready. How could you explain to her the benefits of reducing the number of days her husband is invasively ventilated?

    _____

    _____

    _____

21. What role does NIV play in "end-of-life" situations?

    _____

    _____

    _____

22. List five indications for the use of NIV for adult patients with acute respiratory failure.

    a. _____

    b. _____

    c. _____

    d. _____

    e. _____

23. List the signs and symptoms of respiratory distress in patients who may require ventilatory assistance? Include the arterial blood gas criteria as well.

    _____

    _____

24. You are the respiratory therapist (RT) working in the emergency department (ED) of a level 1 trauma center when a 28-year-old patient is brought in via emergency medical services with a possible head injury. He is confused, tachypneic, tachycardic, and hemodynamically unstable. Would you suggest NIV to the trauma surgeon? Why or why not?

    _____

    _____

    _____

25. What is the final consideration in the selection of patients with acute respiratory failure for NIV?

    _____

    _____

26. What are the physiologic criteria for the institution of NIV for patients with severe stable COPD in a chronic care setting?

    _____

    _____

    _____

27. How do portable pressure-targeted ventilators maintain pressure levels and flush exhaled gases from the circuit?

_____

_____

28. What are the trigger, limit, and cycle variables for bilevel CPAP (BiPAP)?

_____

_____

29. What are the inspiratory and expiratory settings called on the BiPAP?

_____

30. The typical ranges for the inspiratory and expiratory settings on the BiPAP are

_____

31. Most pressure-targeted ventilators offer what modes of ventilatory support?

_____

32. What determines the patient's tidal volume during the use of a pressure-targeted ventilator?

_____

_____

_____

33. Where is the source for unintentional leaks in a pressure-targeted ventilator?

_____

34. What makes the pressure-targeted ventilators able to flow trigger even though there are intentional and unintentional leaks in the system?

_____

35. Explain how average volume assured pressure support (AVAPS) devices work.

_____

_____

_____

36. What patient population may AVAPS be useful?

_____

37. List four factors that cause the F_IO_2 for a portable pressure-targeted ventilator to be variable.

a. _____

b. _____

c. _____

d. _____

38. How can precise oxygen concentrations be delivered through a pressure-targeted ventilator (PTV)?

_____

_____

39. How can CO_2 rebreathing be minimized with a PTV?

_____

_____

40. List the advantages and disadvantages of using an adult acute care ventilator for NIV?

_____

_____

_____

_____

41. When using an adult acute care ventilator for NIV, which mode will make the patient most comfortable and why?

_____

_____

_____

_____

42. Why is it important for heated humidity to be added during NIV?

_____

_____

_____

43. What type of heated humidifier is recommended for NIV? Why?

_____

Chapter **19** **Basic Concepts of Noninvasive Positive-Pressure Ventilation**

44. What advantages does the nasal mask have over the full face mask during the administration of NIV?

_____

_____

_____

_____

45. List two common disadvantages of the nasal mask.

   a. _____

   b. _____

46. What are the major concerns about using the full face mask and total face mask for the administration of NIV?

_____

_____

_____

_____

47. How much dead space volume does a full face mask have?

_____

48. In what position should the patient be when NIV is being initiated?

_____

49. After ensuring proper mask size and fit, what steps should be taken to initiate NIV?

_____

_____

_____

_____

_____

_____

50. What clinical indicators demonstrate improvement in patient comfort?

_____

_____

_____

51. What measures can be taken to ensure patient comfort when the clinical indicators are absent?

_____

_____

_____

52. What tidal volume range should be used with NIV? How is volume manipulated?

_____

_____

_____

_____

53. When should attempts at the use of NIV be terminated in favor of more invasive measures?

_____

_____

_____

54. What factors affect aerosol delivery during NIV?

_____

_____

_____

55. What problems do nasal masks or full face masks present during aerosol delivery?

_____

_____

56. What causes pressure sores on the nasal bridge, and what can be done to alleviate this problem?

_____

_____

_____

_____

57. What can be done to reduce gastric insufflation during NIV?

_____

_____

58. List the five most serious complications of NIV.

   a. _____

   b. _____

   c. _____

   d. _____

   e. _____

59. What are the common methods of weaning a patient from NIV?

   _____

CRITICAL THINKING QUESTIONS

1. Describe a clinical situation that would cause an NIV *not* to trigger from expiratory positive airway pressure (EPAP) to inspiratory positive airway pressure breathing (IPAP) or cycle from IPAP to EPAP?

   _____

   _____

   _____

2. What are the issues that lead to patient noncompliance with NIV, and how can they be alleviated?

   _____

   _____

   _____

3. Describe how placement of the leak port and oxygen bleed-in affects the F_IO_2 delivered to the patient through NIV.

   _____

   _____

   _____

   _____

   _____

   _____

Case Study 1

A 68-year-old male is currently in the ED being seen for what appears to be an exacerbation of congestive heart failure. He is oriented to person, place, and time but is very anxious. Physical examination findings are as follows: pulse 129 beats/min and thready; blood pressure 108/64 mm Hg; temperature 37°C; respirations are 28 breaths/min, shallow, and labored, with accessory muscle use. Auscultation reveals bilateral decreased breath sounds with diffuse coarse crackles on inspiration. The patient has no cough and is diaphoretic. The RT places the patient on a nonrebreather mask and draws an arterial blood gas (ABG) after 15 minutes. The ABG shows pH 7.31, $PaCO_2$ 49 mm Hg, P_aO_2 53 mm Hg, S_aO_2 86%, and HCO_3^- 23 mEq/L.

1. Does this patient meet the selection criteria for NIV? Why or why not?

   _____

   _____

   _____

   _____

2. If NIV is appropriate, what settings should be used? If not, what other respiratory therapy should be initiated?

   _____

   _____

   _____

   _____

After 3 hours of treatment, the patient has become agitated, confused, and uncooperative.

3. What action should be taken at this time?

   _____

   _____

   _____

Case Study 2

A 75-year-old man with a long history of COPD and a past smoking history of 114 pack-years presents to the ED with shortness of breath, productive cough with green purulent sputum, and cyanosis. He has had two prior hospitalizations for acute infective exacerbations of his COPD within the past year. He has no comorbidities or occupational exposure. Physical examination reveals the following: pulse 105 beats/min and regular, blood pressure 140/85 mm Hg, respirations 30 breaths/min with prolonged expiration and use of accessory muscles, percussion is hyper-resonant, breath sounds are reduced bilaterally with prolonged expiratory wheezes. Laboratory work shows white blood cells (WBCs) 11,500 cells/mm^3 and room air ABG pH 7.30, $PaCO_2$ 55 mm Hg, P_aO_2 53 mm Hg, and HCO_3^- 32 mEq/L.

1. Analyze this situation and identify and explain five presenting problems.

   _____

   _____

   _____

   _____

   _____

   _____

2. What treatment recommendations should be suggested for this patient at this time?

   _____

   _____

   _____

   _____

   _____

A repeat ABG following appropriate therapy reveals the following: pH 7.19, $PaCO_2$ 67 mm Hg, P_aO_2 60 mm Hg.

3. What is the most appropriate treatment option at this time?

   _____

   _____

   _____

NBRC-STYLE QUESTIONS

1. Symptoms of chronic hypoventilation include which of the following?
   1. Fatigue
   2. Morning headache
   3. Hypoxemia
   4. Insomnia
   a. 1 and 2 only
   b. 2 and 3 only
   c. 3 and 4 only
   d. 1 and 4 only

2. A male COPD patient, 5 feet 10 inches tall, has been placed on NIV with an IPAP of 8 cm H_2O and an EPAP of 4 cm H_2O. The patient's exhaled volume was measured at 350 mL, and the ABGs on this setting were pH 7.27, $PaCO_2$ 77 mm Hg, P_aO_2 50 mm Hg, and base excess +7. The most appropriate action is which of the following?
   a. Increase EPAP to 6 cm H_2O.
   b. Increase IPAP to 10 cm H_2O.
   c. Decrease IPAP to 6 cm H_2O.
   d. Bleed in 4 L/min of oxygen.

3. The target tidal volume for a patient with an ideal body weight of 58 kg who is receiving NIV is which of the following?
   a. 250 mL
   b. 350 mL
   c. 500 mL
   d. 700 mL

4. The RT notices that there has been a drop in the exhaled tidal volume of a patient receiving NIV. The most appropriate action to take is which of the following?
   a. Increase the IPAP
   b. Decrease the EPAP
   c. Adjust the interface
   d. Change the tubing

5. A patient with chronic hypercapnic respiratory failure is currently using NIV only at night, with the following parameters: assist mode, IPAP 9 cm H_2O, EPAP 4 cm H_2O. The patient is noted to be short of breath with a spontaneous rate of 25 breaths/min. The action that will alleviate this problem is which of the following?
   a. Switch to the control mode.
   b. Increase the IPAP percentage to 35%.
   c. Decrease the EPAP to 2 cm H_2O.
   d. Increase the IPAP to 11 cm H_2O.

Chapter **19** **Basic Concepts of Noninvasive Positive-Pressure Ventilation**

6. Which of the following situations will provide the highest oxygen concentration to a patient who is using a portable pressure-targeted ventilator?
   a. Low IPAP and EPAP settings
   b. High IPAP and EPAP settings
   c. Leak port and oxygen bleed-in at the mask
   d. Leak port and oxygen bleed-in in the circuit

7. The most appropriate type of humidifier to use with NIV is which of the following?
   a. Wick-type humidifier
   b. Heat moisture exchanger
   c. Heated bubble humidifier
   d. Heated passover-type humidifier

8. Which of the following will reduce a significant air leak through the mouth of a patient who is receiving NIV via a nose mask?
   a. Using a chin strap
   b. Adding a forehead spacer
   c. Switching to nasal pillows
   d. Tightening the headgear straps

9. A patient is receiving mask CPAP with 8 cm H_2O and 80% oxygen. The ABG on this setting is pH 7.37, $PaCO_2$ 37 mm Hg, and P_aO_2 55 mm Hg. The most appropriate recommendation is which of the following?
   a. Increase the F_IO_2 to 90%.
   b. Intubate and mechanically ventilate.
   c. Increase the CPAP level to 12 cm H_2O.
   d. Switch to bilevel positive-pressure ventilation.

10. A patient with which of the following problems should be excluded from a trial with NIV?
    a. Amyotrophic lateral sclerosis
    b. Cardiogenic pulmonary edema
    c. Hemodynamically unstable acute respiratory distress syndrome
    d. CAP

20 Weaning and Discontinuation from Mechanical Ventilation

LEARNING OBJECTIVES

Upon completion of this chapter, the reader will be able to do the following:

1. List weaning parameters and the acceptable values for ventilator discontinuation.
2. Compare the three standard modes of weaning in relation to their success in discontinuing ventilation.
3. Define the closed-loop modes of weaning described in the chapter.
4. Recognize appropriate clinical use of closed-loop modes of weaning from a description of a clinical setting.
5. Identify assessment criteria for discontinuing a spontaneous breathing trial in a clinical situation.
6. Describe the criteria used to determine whether a patient is ready for extubation.
7. Recognize postextubation difficulties from a clinical case description.
8. Recommend appropriate treatment for postextubation difficulties.
9. State the first recommendation for weaning a patient from mechanical ventilation, as established by the task force formed by the American College of Chest Physicians, the Society of Critical Care Medicine, and the American Association for Respiratory Care.
10. Describe an appropriate treatment for a patient with an irreversible respiratory disorder that requires long-term ventilation.
11. Name the parameter used as the primary index of drive to breathe.
12. Suggest adjustments to ventilator settings during use of a standard weaning mode, based on patient assessment.
13. Explain the appropriate procedure for management of a patient for whom a spontaneous breathing trial has failed.
14. Defend the use of therapist-driven protocols as key components of efficient and effective patient weaning.
15. Explain the function of long-term care facilities in the management of ventilator-dependent patients.
16. Assess data used to establish the probable cause of failure to wean.

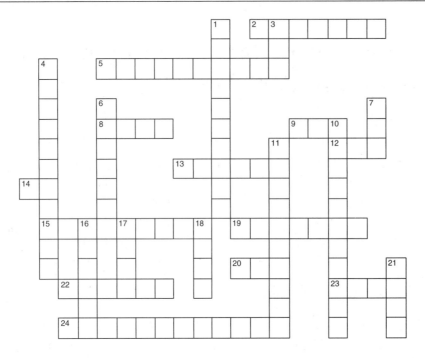

Across

2 Type of epinephrine used to treat airway edema following extubation
5 Area of edema that may occur after the endotracheal tube (ET) is removed
8 The gradual reduction in support
9 A non-physician-directed protocol (abbreviation)
12 A mode designed to make automatic adjustments from the time ventilation is initiated until ventilation can be discontinued (abbreviation)
13 Adapter used during a T-piece weaning from mechanical ventilation
14 Volume-targeted pressure support (abbreviation)
15 Respiratory _____ is the altering use of the diaphragm and accessory muscles to breath
19 A postextubation sound heard when subglottic edema is present
20 Trial of sustained breathing without mechanical support (abbreviation)
22 A low-density gas mixture
23 Index that evaluates compliance, respiratory rate, oxygenation, and inspiratory pressure (abbreviation)
24 Placement of an ET tube following recent removal of it

Down

1 Removal of the ET tube
3 A feature intensive care unit (ICU) ventilators have to deliver exactly the amount of pressure required to overcome the resistive load imposed by the ET (abbreviation)
4 A type of spasm that may occur after the ET tube is removed
6 This psychological factor is high when patients are optimistic and motivated to recover.
7 This can be added to spontaneous breaths to reduce the work of breathing (WOB) (abbreviation)
10 Type of breathing in which the chest wall moves in during inspiration and out during exhalation
11 Associated with a suppressed gag or cough reflex
16 A type of breathing trial
17 Index for ventilatory muscle capability that is calculated using the frequency and tidal volume (abbreviation)
18 This psychological factor is high when patients lie passively in bed
21 Ventilation without an ET (abbreviation)

CHAPTER REVIEW QUESTIONS

1. Define the term *weaning*.

_____

2. Describe three clinical scenarios in which patients typically do not require a slow withdrawal process from mechanical ventilation.

   a. _____

   b. _____

   c. _____

3. List three potential consequences that may be avoided by discontinuing mechanical ventilation as soon as possible.

   a. _____

   b. _____

   c. _____

4. List three potential hazards associated with the premature withdrawal of ventilatory support or of the airway.

   a. _____

   b. _____

   c. _____

5. List three approaches commonly used to reduce ventilatory support.

   a. _____

   b. _____

   c. _____

6. Newer, more sophisticated closed-loop modes used for weaning patients include the following:

   _____

   _____

7. What should be the primary factor in determining whether a patient is ready to be weaned from mechanical ventilation?

   _____

8. Describe the underlying theory of intermittent mandatory ventilation (IMV) that helps facilitate weaning of a patient from mechanical ventilation.

   _____

   _____

9. Why is pressure support (PS) added during IMV?

   _____

   _____

10. What are the trigger, limit, and cycle variables for pressure support ventilation (PSV)?

   _____

   _____

11. What parameters are within the patient's control during PSV?

   _____

12. What is the most practical method of establishing the level of PSV?

   _____

   _____

13. What are considered acceptable ranges for the V_T and respiratory rate for a patient receiving PSV?

   _____

   _____

14. List four signs or symptoms that would indicate an inappropriately set PS level.

   _____

   _____

   _____

15. What is the major disadvantage of T-piece weaning?

   _____

   _____

16. (a) What mode of mechanical ventilation can be used as a substitute for T-piece weaning?

   _____

   (b) What is the major advantage of using this mode instead of a T-piece trial?

   _____

17. In the following list, match the description with the appropriate weaning mode.

Weaning Mode	Description
_____ ATC	(a) Allows spontaneous breathing between mechanical breaths
_____ VS	(b) Similar to a T-piece with alarm support capability
_____ MMV	(c) Compensates for increased resistance and WOB through an ET
_____ ASV	(d) Adjusts to various levels of support automatically
_____ Automode	(e) Allows patient control of the rate, time, and depth of each breath
_____ IMV	(f) Provides pressure-limited breaths that target a volume and rate
_____ PSV	(g) Maintains a consistent minimum minute ventilation
_____ CPAP	(h) Delivers a set VT in a pressure mode of ventilation

18. List three clinical criteria for weaning.

a. _____

b. _____

c. _____

19. List four psychological factors that may adversely affect the weaning process.

a. _____

b. _____

c. _____

d. _____

20. Your patient's total parenteral nutrition was set inappropriately low while receiving mechanical ventilation. What implications does this have on her ability to be weaned from mechanical ventilation?

_____

_____

21. Describe the procedure for a cuff leak test.

_____

_____

22. In a cuff leak test, what does the measured volume that escapes from around a deflated cuff indicate?

_____

_____

23. Why is vital capacity not considered a good indicator for discontinuation of ventilator support?

_____

_____

24. What parameter is a primary index of the inspiratory drive to breathe?

_____

25. A _____ (high; low) oxygen cost of breathing and a (an) _____ (increased; decreased) metabolic rate may result in increased WOB.

26. (a) What index is used to assess the potential for respiratory muscle overload and fatigue?

_____

(b) What four components does this index measure?

1. _____

2. _____

3. _____

4. _____

27. (a) Calculate the index that evaluates compliance, respiratory rate, oxygenation, and inspiratory pressure (CROP index) using these data: C_D = 20 mL/cm H_2O, P_{Imax} = 25 cm H_2O, P_aO_2 = 70 mm Hg, P_AO_2 = 100 mm Hg, rate = 18 breaths/min.

a. _____

b. _____

c. _____

d. _____

(b) Does this value indicate the possibility of successful ventilator withdrawal? Give your reasons.

_____

_____

28. How long must a patient tolerate a spontaneous breathing trial (SBT) to be considered ready for ventilator discontinuation and extubation?

_____

29. What is the formula for the rapid shallow breathing index (RSBI)?

_____

30. Calculate the RSBI, given the following values: V_T = 600 mL, rate = 26 breaths/min.

_____

31. What values of a RSBI indicate that weaning may be successful? _____

32. List the two criteria that must be met before a decision can be made to remove an artificial airway.

    a. _____

    b. _____

33. List four factors that indicate extubation is likely to be successful.

    a. _____

    b. _____

    c. _____

    d. _____

34. List three clinical patient conditions in which an artificial airway should not be removed after weaning from mechanical ventilation.

    a. _____

    b. _____

    c. _____

35. List three complications associated with prolonged intubation.

    a. _____

    b. _____

    c. _____

36. How does administration of heliox aid the treatment of partial airway obstruction and stridor caused by postextubation glottic edema?

_____

_____

37. How is heliox therapy administered in this situation?

_____

38. List six factors that can increase the risk of aspiration after extubation.

    a. _____

    b. _____

    c. _____

    d. _____

    e. _____

    f. _____

39. What is the primary indication for noninvasive positive-pressure ventilation (NIV) after extubation?

_____

_____

40. List five benefits of using NIV after extubation.

    a. _____

    b. _____

    c. _____

    d. _____

    e. _____

41. List the criteria for instituting NIV when an extubated patient is unable to sustain adequate ventilation.

_____

_____

_____

_____

_____

42. List four types of medication that can depress the central ventilatory drive.

    a. _____

    b. _____

    c. _____

    d. _____

43. Explain the advantages of therapist-driven protocols for both patients and hospital staff.

_____

_____

_____

44. List the clinical characteristics of patients that may benefit from a tracheostomy tube placement?

_____

_____

_____

_____

_____

45. List five beneficial outcomes for performing a tracheotomy.

a. _____

b. _____

c. _____

d. _____

e. _____

46. What alternative sites are available for patients who are medically stable, yet still require mechanical ventilation following multiple failed weaning attempts in the ICU?

_____

_____

_____

_____

47. List five goals for weaning in long-term care facilities.

a. _____

b. _____

c. _____

d. _____

e. _____

CRITICAL THINKING QUESTIONS

For Questions 1 and 2, refer to the following scenario.

A patient is successfully weaned from mechanical ventilatory support. A leak test is performed before extubation, and the measured volume is 80 mL.

1. What can the respiratory therapist conclude from this finding?

_____

_____

2. What should the respiratory therapist recommend before extubation?

_____

_____

3. Ten minutes after a patient was extubated, the respiratory therapist hears marked stridor, increased WOB, intercostal retractions, and a 20% drop in the SpO_2. An aerosolized racemic epinephrine treatment is given, but no effect is noted. What should the therapist recommend?

_____

_____

_____

4. You are discussing the best mode of weaning a patient from mechanical ventilation with the attending physician, who prefers to use IMV as a means of weaning patients. You would like to try PSV on this patient. The physician asks you why? Explain why you would choose PSV by comparing and contrasting it to IMV.

_____

_____

CASE STUDIES

Case Study 1

While monitoring a patient 10 minutes after initiation of a T-piece trial through the ventilator, the respiratory therapist observes increased restlessness, an increase in the respiratory rate from 16 to 36 breaths/min, with paradoxical chest movement and use of accessory muscles, and an increase in the heart rate from 80 to 120 beats/min.

1. What may be the primary reason for this patient's failed weaning attempt?

_____

_____

_____

2. What would be the most appropriate action to take at this time?

_____

_____

Case Study 2

A 45-year-old male trauma patient has been maintained on volume-controlled ventilation for approximately 2 weeks. The patient's overall condition is improving, but he is not totally alert, and he has periods of apnea. The physician would like to start weaning the patient from the ventilator.

1. What weaning modalities should the therapist recommend and why?

_____

_____

_____

_____

_____

Case Study 3

A 65-year-old patient who suffered a myocardial infarction several days ago is being ventilated in a volume control mode at a set rate of 12 breaths/min and a V_T of 600 mL. The patient's condition is currently stable, and his overall condition is improving. The physician asks the respiratory therapist to initiate a weaning trial; the results are as follows:

Mode	IMV
Mandatory rate	6 breaths/min
Mandatory V_T	600 mL
Spontaneous rate	35 breaths/min
Spontaneous V_T	185 mL

1. What is the cause of the high spontaneous respiratory rate?

_____

_____

_____

2. What are the therapist's options at this point?

_____

_____

_____

NBRC-STYLE QUESTIONS

1. In the assessment of a patient's respiratory rate, which of the following values would indicate the highest probability that the patient will likely be able to maintain spontaneous ventilation?
   a. Less than 45 breaths/min
   b. Less than 40 breaths/min
   c. Less than 30 breaths/min
   d. Less than 25 breaths/min

2. Which of the following drugs is used most often to treat postextubation glottic edema?
   a. Racemic epinephrine
   b. Intravenous steroids
   c. Albuterol via metered-dose inhaler
   d. Cromolyn sodium

3. Which of the following is the minimal acceptable range for maximal inspiratory pressure when assessing ventilatory muscle strength?
   a. -5 to -10 cm H_2O
   b. -10 to -15 cm H_2O
   c. -20 to -30 cm H_2O
   d. -40 to -50 cm H_2O

4. A patient is being weaned from mechanical ventilation. The ventilator settings and arterial blood gas results are as follows.

Mode	IMV
Set rate	8 breaths/min
V_T	650 mL
F_IO_2	0.35
PS	25 cm H_2O
pH	7.44
$PaCO_2$	34 mm Hg
P_aO_2	96 mm Hg

Based on this information, what should the respiratory therapist recommend?
   a. Increase the synchronized IMV rate
   b. Reduce the PS level
   c. Reduce the V_T
   d. Reduce the F_IO_2

5. Which of the following statements is true?
   a. In IMV, all breaths are spontaneously triggered.
   b. In the A/C mode, every patient effort delivers the set V_T.
   c. In IMV, all breaths deliver the same V_T.
   d. PS can be used to augment the V_T in A/C.

6. A patient is being weaned in the MMV mode. The MMV is set at 7 L, and the patient is breathing at a rate of 14 breaths/min with a spontaneous V_T of 600 mL. How much ventilatory assistance is the ventilator providing?
   a. Minute ventilation of 4 L
   b. No assistance required
   c. Respiratory rate of 8 breaths/min
   d. Minute ventilation of 7 L

7. Which of the following would indicate a successful weaning trial and extubation?
   1. P_aO_2 80 mm Hg on $F_IO_2 \leq 0.4$
   2. P_aO_2/F_IO_2 ratio ≤ 150 to 200 mm Hg
   3. Dopamine greater than 5 mg/kg/min to maintain blood pressure
   4. pH 7.38
   a. 1
   b. 2, 3, and 4
   c. 1 and 4
   d. 1, 2, 3, and 4

8. Which of the following modes of mechanical ventilation automatically adjusts ventilatory parameters based on continuous monitoring of compliance and airway resistance?
   1. Proportional assist ventilation
   2. Pressure-regulated volume control
   3. Adaptive support ventilation
   4. Airway pressure release ventilation
   a. 1 and 2
   b. 1 and 3
   c. 1, 2, and 4
   d. 1, 2, 3, and 4

9. Which of the following should be required before an SBT?
   1. The patient should be given a sedative.
   2. The patient should be able to maintain an adequate P_aO_2 and P_aCO_2 during spontaneous breathing.
   3. The patient should be hemodynamically stable.
   4. The patient's P_{Imax} should be 50 mm Hg.
   a. 1
   b. 1, 2, and 3
   c. 1, 2, 3, and 4
   d. 2 and 3

10. Which of the following parameters indicates that an SBT will likely be successful?
   a. Minute ventilation of 14 L
   b. P_aO_2 of 55 mm Hg on an F_IO_2 of 0.5
   c. V_D/V_T ratio of 0.7
   d. P_aO_2/F_IO_2 ratio of 280 mm Hg

21 Long-Term Ventilation

LEARNING OBJECTIVES

On completion of this chapter, the reader will be able to do the following:

1. State the goals of mechanical ventilation in a home environment.
2. List the criteria for selection of patients suitable for successful home care ventilation.
3. Name the factors used to estimate the cost of home mechanical ventilation.
4. Describe facilities used for the care of patients requiring extended ventilator management in terms of type of care provided and cost.
5. Identify the factors used when considering selection of a ventilator for home use.
6. Compare the criteria for discharging a child versus discharging an adult who is ventilator dependent.
7. Explain the use of the following noninvasive ventilation techniques: pneumobelt, chest cuirass, full-body chamber (tank ventilator), and body suit (jacket ventilator).
8. List follow-up assessment techniques used with home-ventilated patients.
9. Describe some of the difficulties families experience when caring for a patient in the home.
10. Identify pieces of equipment that are essential to accomplishing intermittent positive-pressure ventilation in the home.
11. Name the specific equipment needed for patients in the home who cannot be without ventilator support.
12. Name the appropriate modes used with first-generation portable/home care ventilators.
13. On the basis of a patient's assessment and ventilator parameters, name the operational features required for that patient's home ventilator and any additional equipment that will be needed.
14. Discuss the instructions given to the patient and caregivers when preparing a patient for discharge home.
15. List the items that should appear in a monthly report of patients on home mechanical ventilation.
16. Describe patients who would benefit from continuous positive airway pressure by nasal mask or pillows.
17. Recommend solutions to potential complications and side effects of nasal mask continuous positive airway pressure (CPAP).
18. Recognize from a clinical example a potential complication of negative-pressure ventilation.
19. Name three methods of improving secretion clearance besides suctioning.
20. List the advantages of using mechanical insufflation-exsufflation in conjunction with positive-pressure ventilation.
21. List five psychological problems that can occur in ventilator-assisted individuals (VAIs).
22. Explain the procedure for accomplishing speech in VAIs.
23. Compare the functions of the Portex and the Pitts speaking tracheostomy tubes.
24. Name one essential step required by the respiratory therapist when setting up a speaking valve for a VAI.
25. List six circumstances in which speaking devices may be contraindicated.

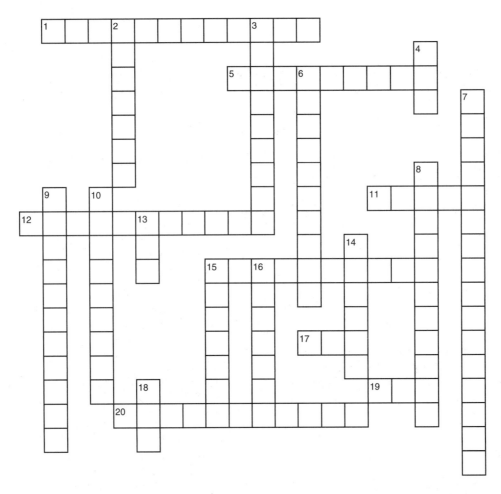

Across

1 Easy to understand and manipulate (two words)
5 Reflux can cause this to erode
11 An obstruction of the intestinal tract associated with immobility of the bowel or a mechanical blockage
12 To remove a tracheostomy tube
15 These must vibrate to produce a voice (two words)
17 Home care equipment supplier (abbreviation)
19 Mechanical cough machine (abbreviation)
20 Type of tube that goes into the stomach

Down

2 Temporary relief for the caregiver
3 Type of planning team
4 Type of sleep disorder (abbreviation)
6 Intermittent abdominal pressure ventilator
7 Type of breathing used to assist patients with poor respiratory muscle strength, also called "frog" breathing
8 Type of tracheostomy tube with an extra opening
9 Surgical opening between the jejunum and the surface of the abdominal wall
10 Type of speaking valve (two words)
13 Opposite of PPV (abbreviation)
14 A speaking tracheostomy tube that has an opening in the posterior portion above the cuff
15 Home care disinfectant
16 Type of ventilation indicated in 13 down
18 Ventilator-assisted individuals (abbreviation)

CHAPTER REVIEW QUESTION

1. List six goals of long-term home or other alternative care site mechanical ventilation.

   a. _____

   b. _____

   c. _____

   d. _____

   e. _____

   f. _____

2. What is considered improvement in psychosocial well-being for a long-term ventilator patient?

   _____

3. How does the American College of Chest Physicians define a long-term ventilator-assisted patient?

   _____

   _____

4. What are the two general categories of patients requiring long-term mechanical ventilation (LTMV)?

   a. _____

   b. _____

5. What are the three patient selection criteria that are assessed when evaluating a patient for home mechanical ventilation?

   a. _____

   b. _____

   c. _____

6. What types of patients are most likely to be successful with long-term ventilation?

   _____

   _____

   _____

   _____

   _____

7. Describe the clinical factors you would assess prior to recommending a patient for LTMV in the home or in a long-term care facility.

   _____

   _____

8. List four additional criteria must be considered for a child to be considered for home mechanical ventilation.

   a. _____

   b. _____

   c. _____

   d. _____

9. Which type of facility would a patient who has required mechanical ventilation for over 30 days and also requires intravenous therapy best be treated?

   _____

10. List six factors that must be considered when estimating a patient's cost of home mechanical ventilation.

    a. _____

    b. _____

    c. _____

    d. _____

    e. _____

    f. _____

11. What is the location that is the least expensive for patients who require long-term ventilatory care?

    _____

12. List the five most important factors when choosing a ventilator for home use.

    a. _____

    b. _____

    c. _____

    d. _____

    e. _____

13. What backup equipment is necessary for a patient requiring LTMV at home? What is the rationale for each?

Backup Equipment	Rationale
_____	_____
_____	_____
_____	_____

14. What is the rationale for the increased level of follow-up and evaluation of the ventilatory status of children maintained on mechanical ventilation at home as compared with adults?

_____

_____

15. Identify three classifications of ventilator-dependent patients.

a. _____

b. _____

c. _____

16. List four psychosocial factors that must be addressed to ensure a successful transition home for the ventilator-dependent patient.

a. _____

b. _____

c. _____

d. _____

17. List five factors that must be addressed when evaluating the home environment prior to discharge of patients requiring mechanical ventilation.

a. _____

b. _____

c. _____

d. _____

e. _____

18. Before a patient is discharged to the home care setting, the primary caregiver asks you what difficulties may be experienced when caring for a patient in the home. How would you respond?

_____

_____

_____

19. In addition to the mechanical ventilator and its related equipment, list six of the other equipment/supplies that are needed to support the patient receiving mechanical ventilation in the home.

a. _____

b. _____

c. _____

d. _____

e. _____

f. _____

20. Before discharge, what are the primary skills the respiratory therapist must teach the patient, his or her family, and others involved in the care of the patient?

_____

_____

_____

21. What components must be included in a written monthly report when performing a home visit?

_____

_____

_____

22. List the three electrical power sources used by home ventilators.

a. _____

b. _____

c. _____

23. List three contraindications for the use of negative-pressure ventilators.

a. _____

b. _____

c. _____

24. Explain why a patient receiving mechanical ventilation with oxygen and positive end-expiratory pressure (PEEP) in the home may encounter difficulty triggering the ventilator.

_____

_____

_____

25. What are some of the advantages of providing home mechanical ventilation with the newer (second-generation) portable home care ventilators?

_____

_____

_____

_____

26. List the four most common gastrointestinal disorders associated with patients receiving LTMV.

a. _____

b. _____

c. _____

d. _____

27. A substantial number of patients who transfer to long-term care facilities on mechanical ventilation have what type of disorders?

_____

28. List three factors that contribute to psychological problems in VAIs.

a. _____

b. _____

c. _____

29. How do the rocking bed and pneumobelt support spontaneous ventilation?

_____

_____

30. What patient conditions are contraindications for use of the rocking bed?

_____

_____

31. What type of patient would benefit from a rocking bed as a form of ventilatory support?

_____

32. In what type of therapy is the phrenic nerve stimulated through surgically implanted electrodes?

_____

33. What happens to a patient with obstructive sleep apnea (OSA) patient during sleep?

_____

_____

34. List three goals of CPAP therapy when used to treat OSA.

a. _____

b. _____

c. _____

35. What patient interfaces are available for delivering CPAP therapy?

_____

_____

36. What are the complications associated with CPAP therapy?

_____

_____

_____

37. What are the physical requirements a patient needs to perform glossopharyngeal breathing?

_____

_____

38. What type of patients benefit from the use of glossopharyngeal breathing?

_____

39. What are the minimum vital capacity and peak cough expiratory flow rate necessary to produce an effective cough?

_____

40. List three techniques that aid in management of secretions for patients with neuromuscular disease.

a. _____

b. _____

c. _____

41. How is assisted coughing performed?

_____

_____

42. What are the advantages of mechanical insufflation-exsufflation (MI-E) compared with tracheal suctioning?

_____

_____

43. In what type of patients is MI-E contraindicated?

_____

_____

44. What type of tracheostomy tube should a therapist recommend for a patient who is unable to speak and at risk of aspiration?

_____

45. What type of tracheostomy tube should a therapist recommend for a patient who has no trouble swallowing and can breathe for long periods of time?

_____

46. In addition to deflating the cuff, what ventilator parameters can be adjusted to help a patient produce speech to or improve speech quality?

_____

_____

47. What are the potential hazards of cuff deflation of VAIs?

_____

48. Before a cuff is deflated to allow for speaking, what should the patient be evaluated for?

_____

49. What devices are available to allow VAIs to speak?

_____

_____

_____

50. How does a Passy-Muir speaking valve allow for speech in the patient with a tracheostomy who is receiving mechanical ventilation?

_____

_____

_____

51. List three clinical circumstances in which the use of speaking devices may be contraindicated.

a. _____

b. _____

c. _____

52. Compare the functions of the Portex and the Pitt speaking tracheostomy tubes.

_____

_____

_____

_____

53. What steps need to be taken prior to setting up a speaking valve for a VAI?

_____

_____

_____

_____

_____

54. What is the most cost-effective disinfecting solution available for home care patients to disinfect their equipment?

_____

55. How long must water be boiled before it can be used in a humidifier?

_____

CRITICAL THINKING QUESTIONS

Questions 1 and 2 refer to the following scenario.

After undergoing a sleep study, a patient diagnosed with OSA is prescribed CPAP via nasal mask. During a follow-up visit by the therapist, the patient states that his sleep is not improving and that he is experiencing eye irritation.

1. What could be the cause of the patient's problem?

_____

_____

2. What steps can the therapist take to alleviate the situation?

_____

_____

Question 3 refers to the following scenario.

A VAI in a long-term [A1]care facility is being maintained on pressure support ventilation. The respiratory therapist is asked to evaluate the patient to see if he can tolerate a speaking valve. After cuff deflation, and before attaching the valve, the patient suddenly becomes short of breath, with an increase in heart rate.

3. What could have brought on the sudden onset of respiratory distress?

_____

_____

_____

_____

Question 4 refers to the following scenario.

Fifteen minutes after initiating PEEP with an external threshold resistor for a patient supported by a home care ventilator, the respiratory therapist observes that the patient's respiratory rate has doubled, her tidal volume has dropped significantly, and the ventilator's low-pressure alarm has been activated.

4. What is the probable cause of this problem?

_____

CASE STUDIES

Case Study 1

A patient in the early stages of a neuromuscular disease complains to his physician that he is having difficulty sleeping. In addition, he is experiencing headaches and becomes increasingly tired toward the end of the day.

1. What are the possible causes of this patient's symptoms?

_____

2. What type of therapy should the therapist recommend to help treat this patient?

_____

3. What would be the goals of the recommended therapy?

_____

4. How would you evaluate the effectiveness of the therapy?

_____

Case Study 2

A 70-year-old female spent 1 month in the hospital for exacerbation of chronic obstructive pulmonary disease (COPD). After numerous attempts at weaning had failed, the patient received a tracheostomy. After careful evaluation, the patient was discharged home on continuous ventilatory support. A follow-up visit was made 2 weeks after discharge. The therapist found the patient to be febrile, auscultation revealed rhonchi in the right upper and middle lobes, and suctioning produced a moderate amount of yellow sputum. The patient was admitted to the hospital and diagnosed with pneumonia.

1. What would be your assessment of why this patient developed a pulmonary infection so soon after discharge?

_____

_____

2. What recommendations, if any, would you make?

_____

_____

NBRC-STYLE QUESTIONS

1. If a home care ventilator does not have an F_IO_2 control, what is the most common means by which oxygen can be delivered to the patient?
   a. Using an external blender
   b. Using a microprocessor-controlled proportioning valve
   c. Mixing air and oxygen cylinders to approximate the desired F_IO_2
   d. Bleeding oxygen into the system through the inspiratory limb

2. In the home setting, how long should suction catheters be soaked in a disinfectant solution?
   a. A minimum of 2 minutes
   b. A minimum of 5 minutes
   c. A minimum of 10 minutes
   d. A minimum of 25 minutes

3. Which of the following represents the range of CPAP levels available on most home care units?
   a. 0 to 2.0 cm H_2O
   b. 2.5 to 20 cm H_2O
   c. 25 to 35 cm H_2O
   d. 35 to 45 cm H_2O

4. Which of the following patient conditions would exclude them from being treated with negative-pressure ventilation?
   a. Excessive secretions
   b. Neuromuscular disease
   c. Spinal cord injuries
   d. Central hypoventilation syndromes

5. During a follow-up visit of a patient recently started on CPAP therapy by nasal mask, the patient complains of nasal dryness and congestion. Which of the following recommendations would help remedy the problem?
   a. Decrease the flow rate
   b. Decrease the level of CPAP
   c. Add humidification or recommend use of a nasal spray
   d. Readjust the mask to correct for any leaks

6. Which of the following is *not* generally part of a monthly home evaluation?
   a. Vital signs
   b. Pulse oximetry
   c. Bedside pulmonary function studies
   d. Arterial blood gas

7. Contraindications to LTMV include the following.
   a. An F_1O_2 requirement greater than 30%
   b. PEEP greater than 5 cm H2O
   c. The need for continuous invasive monitoring
   d. The need for frequent secretion removal

8. Which of the following conditions allow(s) patients certain periods of spontaneous breathing during the day, and generally require(s) only nocturnal ventilatory support?
   1. Myasthenia gravis
   2. End-stage COPD
   3. Kyphoscoliosis
   4. Multiple sclerosis
   a. 1 only
   b. 3 and 4 only
   c. 1, 3, and 4 only
   d. 1, 2, 3, and 4

9. Patient assessment prior to decannulation should include which of the following?
   1. Airway patency
   2. Sufficient muscle strength to generate a cough
   3. Volume and thickness of secretions
   4. Sleep studies
   a. 1 only
   b. 1 and 4 only
   c. 1, 2, and 3 only
   d. 1, 2, 3, and 4

10. Which of the following is not a realistic goal of home mechanical ventilation?
    a. To reverse the disease process
    b. To improve quality of life
    c. To prolong life
    d. To reduce the number of hospitalizations

22 Neonatal and Pediatric Mechanical Ventilation

LEARNING OBJECTIVES

Upon completion of this chapter, the reader will be able to do the following:

1. Discuss the clinical manifestations of respiratory distress in neonatal and pediatric patients.
2. Identify differences in the level of noninvasive ventilatory support.
3. Describe device function and settings for different mechanical respiratory support strategies.
4. Identify the primary and secondary goals of ventilatory support of newborn and pediatric patients.
5. Explain some key areas of assessment that influence the decision on whether to initiate ventilatory support.
6. Recognize the indications, goals, limitations, and potentially harmful effects of continuous positive airway pressure (CPAP) in a clinical case.
7. Describe the basic design of nasal devices used to deliver CPAP to an infant.
8. Compare and contrast a mechanical ventilator equipped with a CPAP delivery system to a freestanding CPAP system.
9. From patient data, recognize the need for mechanical ventilatory support in newborn and pediatric patients.
10. Identify the essential features of a neonatal and pediatric mechanical ventilator.
11. Explain how the advanced features of a ventilator enhance its usefulness over a wide range of clinical settings.
12. Relate the major differences between older generation neonatal ventilators and modern microprocessor-controlled mechanical ventilators.
13. Distinguish demand flow from continuous flow and discuss other modifications that have been made to the basic infant ventilator.
14. Select appropriate ventilator settings based on the patient's weight, diagnosis, and clinical history, and also discuss strategies and rationale for ventilator settings.
15. Discuss newborn and pediatric applications, technical aspects, patient management, and cautions for the following ventilatory modes: pressure-control ventilation (PCV), volume-control ventilation, dual-controlled ventilation, pressure-support ventilation (PSV), airway pressure release ventilation (APRV), and neurally adjusted ventilatory assist (NAVA).
16. Discuss the rationale and indications for high-frequency ventilation (HFV) in newborn and pediatric patients.
17. Compare the characteristics and basic delivery systems of the following HFV techniques: high-frequency positive-pressure ventilation, high-frequency jet ventilation, high-frequency flow interruption, high-frequency percussive ventilation, and high-frequency oscillatory ventilation (HFOV).
18. Explain the physiologic and theoretic mechanisms of gas exchange that govern HFV, and defend the mechanism believed to be most correct.
19. Explain how settings of a given high-frequency technique are initially adjusted, the effect of individual controls on gas exchange, and strategies of patient management.
20. Discuss the physiologic benefits of inhaled nitric oxide (NO) therapy, and suggest recommended treatment strategies.

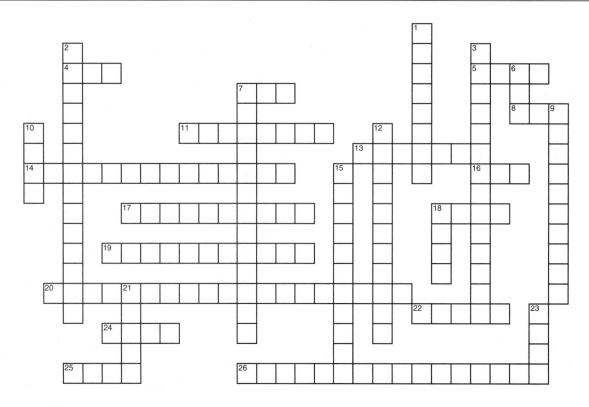

Across

4 Condition that is responsive to 24 across (abbreviation)
5 Type of ventilation that uses the highest rates (8 to 20 Hz) (abbreviation)
7 Pulmonary disease of infants; high airway resistance is a major component (abbreviation)
8 Neonatal problem commonly treated with methylxanthines (abbreviation)
11 Type of aspiration syndrome that occurs in term or post-term neonates
13 Abnormal tube-like passage between the trachea and the esophagus
14 A deficiency in the cartilage around a bronchus; leads to atelectasis
16 Infant who weighs 1500 to 2500 g (abbreviation)
17 Type of heart disease present at birth
18 Mode that is unique to infant mechanical ventilation (abbreviation)
19 Congenital split of the roof of the mouth (two words)
20 Incomplete embryologic formation of the diaphragm leads to this (two words)
22 Type of hemoglobin present in a fetus
24 Noninvasive method of increasing functional residual capacity (FRC) and improving lung compliance
25 Mode of ventilation used to percuss the chest to remove secretions (abbreviation)
26 Structure that may remain open after birth (two words)

Down

1 Trade name for beractant (a surfactant)
2 Softening of the cartilages of the trachea
3 Failure of the nasopharyngeal (NP) septum to rupture causes this malformation (two words)
6 This sleep disorder is usually treated by 24 across (abbreviation)
7 Viral infection that causes inflammation, swelling, and airway obstruction
9 Exchange of gas between lung units with different time constants
10 Infant weighing less than 1500 g (abbreviation)
12 A selective pulmonary vasodilator used to improve pulmonary blood flow and enhance arterial oxygenation (two words)
15 Interface most often used for application of CPAP (two words)
18 Historically, the mode most often used for infants (abbreviation)
21 Mode that uses frequencies up to 150 breaths/min (abbreviation)
23 An invasive life support procedure (abbreviation)

CHAPTER REVIEW QUESTIONS

1. List the three basic types of devices involved in the mechanical ventilation of newborn and pediatric patients.

   a. _____

   b. _____

   c. _____

2. What concepts must a clinician taking care of the neonatal and pediatric population understand?

   _____

   _____

   _____

3. Define the term *respiratory failure*.

   _____

4. Respiratory failure in a neonate is characterized by what laboratory and clinical data?

   _____

   _____

   _____

   _____

5. List the five factors that make neonatal and pediatric patients more vulnerable to rapid deterioration.

   a. _____

   b. _____

   c. _____

   d. _____

   e. _____

6. List four signs or respiratory distress in the neonate.

   a. _____

   b. _____

   c. _____

   d. _____

7. Explain *grunting* in a neonatal patient.

   _____

   _____

   _____

   _____

8. How can tissue oxygenation be assessed physically?

   _____

   _____

   _____

9. In what way can oxygen delivery and tissue perfusion be evaluated clinically?

   _____

10. Give two examples of times when a very individualized approach for managing gas exchange during ventilatory support is needed early in the patient's management.

    a. _____

    b. _____

11. List the five goals of mechanical ventilatory support in newborn and pediatric patients.

    a. _____

    b. _____

    c. _____

    d. _____

    e. _____

12. What are the goals of maintaining an appropriate FRC in a newborn or pediatric patient?

    _____

    _____

13. What laboratory data define respiratory failure in newborns?

    _____

14. The minimum acceptable pH for a premature or term newborn is _____.

15. What laboratory data defines respiratory failure in pediatric patients?

    _____

    _____

16. When maximum oxygen delivery to the tissues is critical, why is fetal hemoglobin not desirable?

    _____

    _____

    _____

17. List the two most common uses for CPAP in pediatric patients.

a. _____

b. _____

18. List four clinical situations in which CPAP would be indicated for a neonatal patient.

a. _____

b. _____

c. _____

d. _____

19. List eight indications for CPAP in the neonate.

a. _____

b. _____

c. _____

d. _____

e. _____

f. _____

g. _____

h. _____

20. List six factors that constitute the physical examination indicators for the use of CPAP.

a. _____

b. _____

c. _____

d. _____

e. _____

f. _____

21. What are the blood gas values that indicate a need for CPAP?

_____

_____

22. List two findings on chest radiograph that may indicate the need for CPAP.

a. _____

b. _____

23. List five conditions that are thought to respond to CPAP and which are associated with one or more of the previously listed clinical presentations.

a. _____

b. _____

c. _____

d. _____

e. _____

24. What are the two general approaches used to minimize the use of mechanical ventilation and protect the neonatal respiratory system?

a. _____

b. _____

25. What does InSURE stand for?

_____

26. List two clinical situations where CPAP therapy can be dangerous to an infant.

a. _____

b. _____

27. When may infants require intubation and mechanical ventilation rather than CPAP?

_____

_____

_____

_____

28. List three methods of delivering CPAP to newborns.

a. _____

b. _____

c. _____

29. What are the most critical facts concerning the application of CPAP interfaces?

_____

_____

30. What should CPAP stabilizing equipment be periodically checked for?

_____

_____

_____

31. List the five components that make up a CPAP system.

   a. _____

   b. _____

   c. _____

   d. _____

   e. _____

32. List four problems that improper positioning of the nasopharyngeal (NP) tube can cause.

   a. _____

   b. _____

   c. _____

   d. _____

33. How is pressure regulated in bubble CPAP machines?

   _____

   _____

34. What is the initial pressure setting for CPAP and how should the CPAP level be adjusted?

   _____

   _____

35. What is considered an adequate level of CPAP?

   _____

   _____

36. List 10 possible complications of CPAP.

   a. _____

   b. _____

   c. _____

   d. _____

   e. _____

   f. _____

   g. _____

   h. _____

   i. _____

   j. _____

37. List four complications that accompany neonatal endotracheal intubation.

   a. _____

   b. _____

   c. _____

   d. _____

38. List four uses of noninvasive positive-pressure ventilation (NIV).

   a. _____

   b. _____

   c. _____

   d. _____

39. Suggested initial intermittent mandatory ventilation settings for neonates.

   _____

   _____

   _____

   _____

40. Describe SiPAP and list the common settings.

   _____

   _____

   _____

41. What are the benefits of bilevel positive airway pressure (BiPAP) and NIV in the pediatric population?

   _____

42. Suggest initial settings for a pediatric patient receiving BiPAP.

   _____

   _____

   _____

43. List four major categories of indications for mechanical ventilation in the neonate.

    a. _____

    _____

    b. _____

    _____

    c. _____

    _____

    d. _____

    _____

44. List seven diseases/syndromes that can reduce lung compliance and/or increase airway resistance in a neonate.

    a. _____

    b. _____

    c. _____

    d. _____

    e. _____

    f. _____

    g. _____

45. List four diseases/syndromes that impair the cardiovascular function of a neonate.

    a. _____

    b. _____

    c. _____

    d. _____

46. List five indications for mechanical ventilation of pediatric patients.

    a. _____

    b. _____

    c. _____

    d. _____

    e. _____

47. What are the arterial blood gas indicators of respiratory failure in pediatric patients?

    _____

    _____

48. In the past, the modality that was used more than any other to ventilate infants was

    _____.

49. In an infant ventilator, what type of trigger avoids breath stacking and asynchrony?

    _____

50. Discuss the difference between continuous flow and demand flow for spontaneous breaths.

    _____

    _____

51. What triggering methods are available for neonatal and pediatric patients?

    _____

    _____

52. What is the preferred triggering method for neonates? Why?

    _____

    _____

53. What is the major limitation of proximal flow sensors?

    _____

54. Describe how peak inspiratory pressure (PIP) can be optimized during manual ventilation.

    _____

    _____

55. What is the purpose of positive end-expiratory pressure (PEEP)?

    _____

56. What are acceptable initial PEEP settings?

    _____

57. When should PEEP be increased?

_____

_____

58. What is meant by the term *flow chop*?

_____

_____

59. (a) Calculate the time constant when R_{aw} = 45 cm/ H_2O/L/s and C_L = 0.004 L/cm H_2O.

_____

_____

   (b) What T_I should be set for this time constant?

_____

60. (a) Calculate the time constant when R_{aw} = 30 cm/ H_2O/L/s and C_L = 0.002 L/cm H_2O.

_____

_____

   (b) What T_I should be set for this time constant?

_____

61. What can be done to reduce the potential for ventilator-induced hyperinflation in patients with bronchopulmonary dysplasia or meconium aspiration?

_____

_____

62. What is considered an acceptable leak around a cuffless endotracheal tube (ET)?

_____

63. Mean airway pressures greater than _____

   have been associated with lung injury in neonates.

64. What P_aO_2 levels should be maintained in neonates and pediatric patients?

_____

_____

65. What parameter is set to ensure a tidal volume during volume-targeted ventilation?

_____

66. What factors determine T_I when volume ventilation is used?

_____

_____

67. What types of pediatric patients respond well to volume controlled-intermittent mandatory ventilation?

_____

_____

68. The recommended V_T values for PSV are

_____.

69. What is a cycling problem that can occur during PSV in patients with an ET or tracheostomy tube?

_____

70. Explain how volume assured pressure support (VAPS) works.

_____

_____

_____

_____

71. What advantage does volume support ventilation (VSV) have over PSV in the administration of surfactant replacement therapy to an infant?

_____

_____

_____

72. How are the pressure levels set in APRV for neonatal and pediatric patients?

_____

_____

73. What benefits does spontaneous breathing at the higher pressure level during APRV provide?

_____

_____

74. What parameters does NAVA allow the patient to control?

_____

_____

75. What are the goals of lung-protective therapy in the neonatal and pediatric patient?

_____

_____

_____

76. When should HFV be considered in an infant's clinical course?

_____

_____

_____

_____

77. List three complications from HFV.

a. _____

b. _____

c. _____

78. Explain the physiologic mechanism of gas exchange in HFV.

_____

_____

79. List the preparations that should be completed before a patient is placed on HFV.

_____

_____

_____

80. What is the general goal for all types of HFV?

_____

_____

81. What do preparations of exogenous surfactant typically contain?

_____

_____

82. Describe the dosing procedure for exogenous surfactant.

_____

_____

_____

_____

_____

_____

83. Name the two types of toxicity that have been reported with application of inhaled NO.

a. _____

b. _____

CRITICAL THINKING QUESTIONS

1. A pediatric patient with a 4-mm ET is receiving PSV. The respiratory therapist notes that inspiration seems to exceed 1 second. What is the most likely cause of this problem and how can it be corrected?

_____

_____

2. VSV has what advantage over PSV during surfactant replacement therapy?

_____

_____

3. An infant receiving nasal CPAP is crying, and each time the infant's mouth opens, the CPAP level on the pressure manometer drops significantly. Why is the pressure dropping and what can be done to correct it?

_____

_____

_____

4. What circumstance can reduce the level of support provided in pressure-regulated volume control? What problems can this lead to?

_____

Case Study 1

A 29 weeks' gestation, 2-hour-old infant is in the neonatal intensive care unit (ICU) in an oxyhood with an F_IO_2 of 0.5. Physical examination reveals intercostal and substernal retractions, a respiratory rate of 68 breaths/min, and a pulse of 145. The arterial blood gas (ABG) values are as follows: pH = 7.21, P_aCO_2 = 70 mm Hg, P_aO_2 = 41 mm Hg. Manual ventilation of this patient demonstrates bilateral chest movement and aeration at 25 cm H_2O.

1. The most appropriate PIP setting for this patient is

_____ .

During mechanical ventilation, the patient's pressure-volume loop changes from that shown in Figure 22-1, *A*, to that shown in Figure 22-1, *B*.

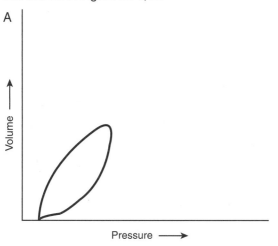

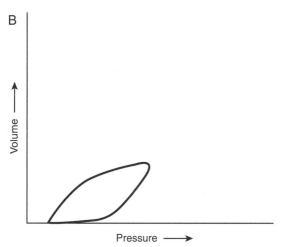

2. What is the most likely cause of this change?

_____

The patient receives Survanta at 2 mL/kg. During this time the ventilator F_IO_2 is increased to 1. Each partial dose is followed by a 30-second period on the ventilator. The pressure-volume loop then takes on the shape shown in Figure 22-2.

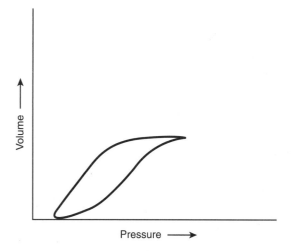

3. What is the most likely cause of this change?

_____

Case Study 2

A newborn male infant weighing 1275 g and approximately 28 weeks' gestation is intubated and receiving mechanical ventilation with time-cycled pressure limited (TCPL) at these settings: rate = 40 breaths/min, PIP = 24 cm H_2O, PEEP = 4 cm H_2O, F_IO_2 = 0.75. The patient received Survanta about 1 hour ago. The ABG results after surfactant therapy were as follows: pH = 7.36, $PaCO_2$ = 38 mm Hg, P_aO_2 = 80 mm Hg. The infant is pink and active; the pulse oximeter reads 96%.

1. What would be the most appropriate action in this situation?

_____

Over the next 2 hours, the patient's oxygen saturations begin to decline and his oxygen requirements increase. Breath sounds are bilaterally diminished, the pulse oximeter reading is 86% with an F_IO_2 of 0.55, and the patient is agitated. The respiratory therapist suctions the patient, but no improvement is noted.

2. Name the two most likely causes of this patient's distress.

_____

_____

3. What is the most appropriate action at this time?

_____

_____

Chapter **22 Neonatal and Pediatric Mechanical Ventilation**

Case Study 3

A 24 weeks' gestation neonate weighing 730 g had no signs of respirations and had central cyanosis at birth. He was intubated in the delivery room and transported to the neonatal ICU. He had poor gas exchange during manual resuscitation, and the decision was made to place him on HFOV.

1. What should be the setting for the mean airway pressure?

   _____

2. The initial frequency setting should be _____ Hertz.

3. How should the initial pressure gradient be set?

   _____

NBRC-STYLE QUESTIONS

1. Which of the following is the best method of ensuring an effective CPAP system?
   a. Use of audible and visual alarm systems
   b. Incorporation of F_IO_2 and pressure monitors
   c. Careful monitoring of the patient's work of breathing and oxygenation status
   d. Use only of a mechanical ventilator with continuous flow capability

2. The type of CPAP delivery system that produces vibrations that may have a beneficial effect is which of the following?
   a. Bubble CPAP
   b. Freestanding CPAP device
   c. Mechanical ventilators with CPAP settings
   d. Improvised freestanding CPAP delivery device

3. The safest and most effective method of CPAP delivery to a newborn is with which of the following?
   a. Vapotherm
   b. Hamilton Arabella
   c. Fisher & Paykel bubble CPAP
   d. Improvised freestanding CPAP device

4. In newborns, PEEP is used to accomplish which of the following?
   1. Recruit alveoli
   2. Prevent atelectasis
   3. Decrease compliance
   4. Establish functional residual capacity
   a. 1 and 3
   b. 1 and 2
   c. 3 and 4
   d. 2 and 4

5. The disease state that prolongs time constants is which of the following?
   a. Acute lung injury
   b. Apnea of prematurity
   c. Bronchopulmonary dysplasia
   d. Respiratory distress syndrome

6. A neonate receiving nasal CPAP of 8 cm H_2O with an F_IO_2 of 0.65 has the following ABG values: pH = 7.2, $PaCO_2$ = 69 mm Hg, and P_aO_2 = 48 mm Hg. The most appropriate action is which of the following?
   a. Increase the F_IO_2 to 0.75
   b. Increase CPAP to 10 cm H_2O
   c. Change to NP CPAP
   d. Intubate and mechanically ventilate with pressure controlled-intermittent mandatory ventilation (PC-IMV)

7. Before an infant is put on PC-IMV, which of the following methods should determine the PIP?
   a. Estimate the PIP for the patient, set the value at a level higher than this, and adjust downward
   b. Compare chest movement and bilateral aeration to the PIP during manual ventilation
   c. Estimate the PIP for the patient, set the value at a level lower than this, and adjust upward as needed
   d. Set the PIP to a safe level, attach the patient to the ventilator, and monitor for improvement in overall appearance and oxygen saturation

8. Calculate the patient's estimated V_T in PC-IMV when T_I is 0.5 second and flow is 8.75 L/min.
   a. 54 mL
   b. 62 mL
   c. 73 mL
   d. 95 mL

9. V_T is increased during PCV by which of the following?
   a. Increasing PIP
   b. Increasing PEEP
   c. Decreasing flow rate
   d. Increasing T_I

10. Which of the following must be monitored during administration of surfactant replacements?
    1. Heart rate
    2. Oxygenation
    3. Temperature
    4. Airway patency
    a. 1, 2, and 4
    b. 2, 3, and 4
    c. 1 and 3
    d. 1, 2, 3, and 4

23 | Special Techniques in Ventilatory Support

LEARNING OBJECTIVES

Upon completion of this chapter, the reader will be able to do the following:

1. Discuss the benefits and disadvantages of airway pressure release ventilation (APRV).
2. Recommend initial settings for initiating APRV in patients with acute respiratory distress syndrome (ARDS).
3. Explain how the controls operate with the SensorMedics 3100B oscillator.
4. Recommend initial ventilator settings for an adult with the 3100B unit.
5. List types of medications that may be used in transitioning from volume-control continuous mandatory ventilation (VC-CMV) to high-frequency oscillatory ventilation (HFOV) for an adult.
6. Explain how the chest wiggle factor is influenced by HFOV settings.
7. Name pulmonary pathologic conditions in which heliox therapy may be beneficial.
8. Compare the differences between set tidal volume (V_T,) monitored V_{TT}, and actual V_T delivery during heliox therapy.
9. Describe how heliox used with a mechanical ventilator may affect pressures and fractional inspired oxygen concentration (F_IO_2) monitoring and delivery.
10. Explain the procedure for using heliox cylinders with a mechanical ventilator.
11. Name at least four techniques that can help determine the correct placement of the esophageal electrical activity of the diaphragm (EDI) catheter.
12. Provide examples of how the EDI waveform can be of value in monitoring critically ill patients.
13. Discuss various factors that can cause a low EDI signal and a high EDI signal.
14. Describe the safety backup features and alarms available with neutrally adjusted ventilator assist (NAVA).
15. Calculate an estimated pressure delivery when given the NAVA level, EDI peak, EDI minimum, and positive end-expiratory pressure (PEEP).
16. Explain what parameters (pressure, flow, volume, and neural signal, time) are used to deliver a breath during NAVA ventilation.
17. Identify clinical situations in which NAVA should be used.

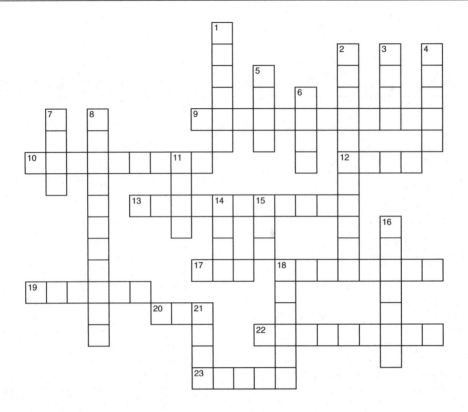

Across

9 Region of the lung that receives the most ventilation
10 HFOV control that influences P_aCO_2
12 Mode of ventilation with two levels of continuous positive airway pressure (CPAP) (abbreviation)
13 Factor observed from the level of the clavicle to the mid-thigh during HFOV (two words)
17 HFOV's equivalent to PEEP (abbreviation)
18 First parameter set in starting HFOV (two words)
19 Helium-oxygen mixture
20 Technique that allows the gas flow to each lung to be controlled separately (abbreviation)
22 Region of the lung receiving the most blood flow
23 A property of helium

Down

1 Forward and backward excursion of this device helps determine V_T
2 Type of breathing allowed during biphasic CPAP
3 Type of flow waveform produced by HFOV
4 Cycles per minute
5 HFOV is used in the management of this pulmonary problem (abbreviation)
6 HFOV control that directly affects P_aO_2 (abbreviation)
7 Heart-lung bypass machine (abbreviation)
8 Brief interval at P_{low} (two words)
11 Type of endotracheal tube (ET) used to accomplish 20 across (abbreviation)
14 Repair of this may cause unilateral lung injury (abbreviation)
15 Applies internal percussion to the lungs (abbreviation)
16 Biphasic CPAP on the Covidien Puritan Bennett 840 (two words)
18 Biphasic CPAP on the SERVO-i (two words)
21 This can be avoided by starting HFOV early in patients with severe ALI/ARDS (abbreviation)

CHAPTER REVIEW QUESTIONS

1. Define *APRV*.

   _____

   _____

   _____

   _____

2. Refer to the APRV waveform in the following figure.

   (a) What is the P_{low}? _____

   (b) What is the P_{high}? _____

   (c) What is the T_{low}? _____

   (d) What is the T_{high}? _____

3. In APRV, what are the trigger and cycle variables when the patient does not breathe?

   _____

4. List two other names for APRV that are used in the United States.

   a. _____

   b. _____

5. List four of the physiologic or hemodynamic advantages of APRV compared with other forms of ventilation.

   a. _____

   b. _____

   c. _____

   d. _____

6. List four disadvantages of APRV.

   a. _____

   b. _____

   c. _____

   d. _____

7. Calculate the APRV respiratory rate that would deliver a P_{low} for 0.75 second and a P_{high} for 4.75 seconds.

   _____

   _____

   _____

8. In APRV, minute ventilation depends on what two factors?

   _____

   _____

9. The range for the P_{high} setting is _____.

10. Why does the practitioner want to set the P_{low} setting at 0 cm H_2O?

    _____

11. The range for the T_{high} setting is _____.

12. How should the T_{low} setting be chosen?

    _____

    _____

    _____

13. For a patient with ARDS, the typical range for the T_{low} setting is _____.

14. List the three factors that determine ventilation and $PaCO_2$ in APRV.

    a. _____

    b. _____

    c. _____

15. Describe one method of weaning a patient from APRV.

    _____

    _____

    _____

    _____

16. HFOV oscillates the lungs at what rates?

    _____

17. What creates the high-frequency oscillations in the SensorMedics 3100B?

_____

18. What determines V_T during HFOV?

_____

_____

19. What determines the appropriateness of the power setting?

_____

_____

20. Increasing the HFOV frequency does what to patient ventilation? Explain.

_____

21. Reducing the HFOV frequency does what to patient ventilation? Explain.

_____

22. What does the $T_I\%$ represent on the SensorMedics 3100B?

_____

_____

23. How does the bias flow setting influence the patient's $PaCO_2$?

_____

_____

_____

24. List the indications for HFOV in adults.

_____

_____

_____

_____

25. What is the one exclusion criterion for use of the SensorMedics 3100B?

_____

26. List the types of medications that may be used in transitioning from VC-CMV to HFOV in an adult.

_____

_____

27. A patient on HFOV may be checked for a return to conventional ventilation when what two parameters have been reached?

_____

28. Describe the physical characteristics of helium.

_____

_____

29. List the pulmonary pathologies that may be treated with heliox therapy.

_____

_____

30. Calculate the actual flow reading for an 80:20 heliox mixture with a displayed flow rate of 6 L/min.

_____

_____

31. Complete the following table, which compares volumes delivered during heliox therapy provided by critical care ventilators.

Ventilator	Volume with Heliox
CareFusion AVEA	_____
Hamilton Veolar and Hamilton Galileo	_____
Covidien Puritan Bennett 840	_____
Servo-i	_____
Drager Dura-2	_____
Drager E-4	_____

32. How is heliox connected to a mechanical ventilator?

_____

_____

33. How does the use of heliox with a mechanical ventilator affect F_IO_2 monitoring?

_____

_____

_____

_____

_____

34. How does the use of heliox with a mechanical ventilator affect pressures?

_____

_____

35. Name a circumstance in which heliox therapy should not be used.

_____

_____

36. What is independent lung ventilation and how is it accomplished?

_____

_____

_____

_____

37. List the surgical procedures in which lung isolation and independent lung ventilation (ILV) are used.

_____

_____

_____

38. Compare synchronous with dyssynchronous ventilation when two ventilators are used for ILV.

_____

_____

_____

_____

_____

_____

39. Define the expiratory inflection point. What is another term used to describe it?

_____

_____

_____

40. What should the mode, rate, and V_T be for performing a less hemodynamically stressful slow-flow inflection maneuver to one lung? To both lungs?

_____

_____

41. How are appropriate levels of PEEP established for each lung during ILV?

_____

_____

_____

42. How is ventilator triggering established during NAVA?

_____

_____

43. List two backup modes set when a patient is being ventilated in the NAVA mode.

_____

_____

44. List five conditions that would exclude a patient from the use of the NAVA mode.

a. _____

b. _____

c. _____

d. _____

e. _____

CRITICAL THINKING QUESTIONS

1. What ventilator mode and settings are represented by the following pressure-time graph?

_____

_____

2. After an adult patient is placed on HFOV, a chest radiograph shows the diaphragm in the midclavicular line to be at the level of the sixth posterior rib. Which ventilator parameter, if any, needs to be changed and why?

_____

_____

For Questions 3 through 5, refer to the pressure-volume curve for a slow-flow inflection maneuver displayed in the following figure.

3. Plot the lower inflection point and the upper inflection point for the static pressure-volume loop.

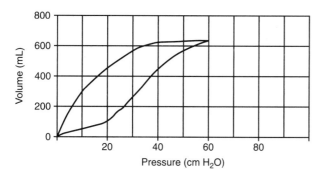

_____

4. PEEP should be set at what level?

_____

5. What V_T should be used to ventilate this patient?

_____

CASE STUDIES

Case Study 1

A patient is ventilated with APRV at the following settings: P_{high} = 20 cm H_2O, P_{low} = 2 cm H_2O, T_{high} = 4 seconds, T_{low} = 1 second, F_IO_2 = 0.4. The patient's spontaneous rate is 12 breaths/min. The current arterial blood gas (ABG) values include a P_aO_2 of 86 mm Hg and a $PaCO_2$ of 68 mm Hg.

1. Calculate the current ventilator rate.

_____

_____

2. Which parameter needs to be changed to correct this patient's problem?

_____

3. State the reason for changing that parameter.

_____

_____

Case Study 2

A patient currently is ventilated with APRV at the following settings: P_{high} = 35 cm H_2O, P_{low} = 5 cm H_2O, T_{high} = 7 seconds, T_{low} = 0.5 second, F_IO_2 = 0.3. The patient's spontaneous rate is 14 breaths/min. The current ABG values include a P_aO_2 of 58 mm Hg and a $PaCO_2$ of 42 mm Hg.

1. Which parameter needs to be changed to correct this patient's problem?

_____

2. State the reason for changing that parameter.

_____

_____

3. If changing the above parameter does not correct this patient's problem, what other change could be made?

_____

_____

Case Study 3

A male patient, 6 feet 2 inches tall and weighing 81 kg, underwent thoracoabdominal surgical repair of an aortic aneurysm and has been brought to the surgical intensive care unit. He is intubated with a double-lumen ET tube, and two ventilators are ready at the bedside.

1. Which lung will have sustained injury as a result of the surgery? Why?

_____

_____

_____

2. What volume should be used in this patient to perform a single-lung slow inflation maneuver to determine inflection points?

_____

3. If the right lung's lower inflection point is 6 cm H_2O and the left lung's lower inflection point is 18 cm H_2O, what is the appropriate PEEP level for each lung?

_____

_____

Chapter **23** **Special Techniques in Ventilatory Support**

1. The advantages of APRV over other forms of conventional ventilation are mainly the result of which of the following?
   a. Preservation of spontaneous breathing
   b. Reduced risk of ventilator-induced lung injury
   c. Reduced risk of ventilator-associated pneumonia
   d. Reduced need for patient sedation and paralysis

2. Which of the following are the most appropriate APRV settings for an ARDS patient who is receiving VC-CMV at these settings: rate $= 12$ breaths/min, $V_T = 600$ mL, $F_1O_2 = 1$, PEEP $= 10$ cm H_2O, peak inspiratory pressure $= 32$ cm H_2O, $P_{plateau} = 25$ cm H_2O?
   a. $P_{high} = 42$ cm H_2O, $P_{low} = 10$ cm H_2O, $T_{high} = 2$ seconds, $T_{low} = 2$ seconds
   b. $P_{high} = 25$ cm H_2O, $P_{low} = 10$ cm H_2O, $T_{high} = 4$ seconds, $T_{low} = 2$ seconds
   c. $P_{high} = 25$ cm H_2O, $P_{low} = 0$, $T_{high} = 4$ seconds, $T_{low} = 1$ second
   d. $P_{high} = 15$ cm H_2O, $P_{low} = 0$, $T_{high} = 6$ seconds, $T_{low} = 1.5$ seconds

3. The parameter that can generally improve oxygenation during APRV is which of the following?
   a. Phigh
   b. Plow
   c. Thigh
   d. T_{low}

4. Calculate the APRV ventilator rate when T_{high} is 12 seconds and T_{low} is 2 seconds.
   a. 4 cycles/min
   b. 6 cycles/min
   c. 9 cycles/min
   d. 12 cycles/min

5. The first parameter set when starting HFOV is which of the following?
   a. $T_1\%$
   b. Frequency
   c. Amplitude
   d. Bias flow

6. A decrease in chest wiggle during HFOV may be caused by which of the following?
   1. Pneumothorax
   2. ET obstruction
   3. Increased $PaCO_2$
   4. Patient improvement
   a. 1 and 2
   b. 2 and 3
   c. 4
   d. 1 and 3

7. An ARDS patient is receiving HFOV at the following settings: $P_{aw} = 28$ cm H_2O, frequency $= 6$ Hz, bias flow $= 30$ L/min, $\Delta P = 7$ (amplitude 60 cm H_2O), $T_1\% = 33$, $F_1O_2 = 0.8$. The patient's P_aO_2 on these settings is 75 mm Hg. Which of the following is the most appropriate action in this case?
   a. Increase the F_1O_2 to 0.9.
   b. Reduce the control to 5.
   c. Reduce the frequency to 5 Hz.
   d. Increase the P_{aw} to 30 cm H_2O.

8. With HFOV, the first step in reducing an adult patient's $PaCO_2$ is which of the following?
   a. Increase the $T_1\%$.
   b. Reduce the frequency.
   c. Increase the amplitude.
   d. Increase the cuff leak.

9. To achieve a flow of 8 L/min for a 70:30 heliox mixture, the oxygen flowmeter should be set at which of the following?
   a. 5 L/min
   b. 8 L/min
   c. 11 L/min
   d. 14 L/min

10. During ventilation with heliox mixtures, most ventilators have which of the following problems?
    1. Inaccurate PEEP measurements
    2. Discrepancies in flow measurements
    3. Discrepancies between the set and actual F_1O_2
    4. Nonlinear relationship between $V_T$set and $V_T$del
    a. 1 and 2
    b. 2 and 3
    c. 3 and 4
    d. 1 and 4

11. An adult patient has a left-sided flail chest and underlying left lung contusions from a motor vehicle accident. The most appropriate mode of ventilation for this patient is which of the following?
    a. ILV
    b. APRV
    c. HFOV
    d. Pressure-controlled ventilation with heliox

12. With HFOV, volume delivery from the oscillator is determined by all of the following except:
    a. $T_1\%$
    b. Oscillator displacement
    c. ET tube size
    d. Patient's ability to trigger the ventilator